exercises
to improve your
HEALTH

Choose the right body moves to improve your health and prevent illness

from asthma and arthritis
to diabetes and high blood pressure

DEBRA DALEY

KT-376-933

CICO BOOKS
LONDON NEW YORK

Published in 2011 by CICO Books
An imprint of Ryland Peters & Small Ltd
20–21 Jockey's Fields
London WC1R 4BW

www.cicobooks.com

10 9 8 7 6 5 4 3 2 1

A CIP catalogue record for this book is available from the
British Library.

ISBN: 978 1907563 69 0

Printed in China

Editor: Marion Paull
Designer: Roger Hammond

Safety Note
Please note that the information in this book should
not be substituted for advice from your physician. If you
have any health concerns, consult your physician for
guidance before doing any of the exercises in this book.
The publisher and author take no responsibility for any
health issue that may arise indirectly or directly from the
use of this book.

Contents

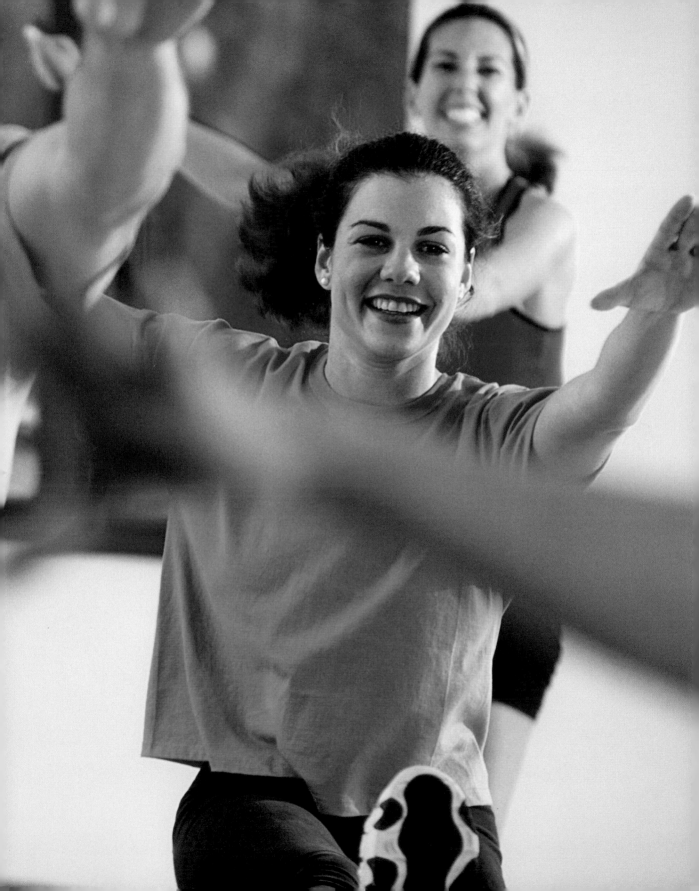

Feel better—live longer

My mother suffered from angina. That's the chest pains a person gets when their heart muscle is low on oxygen-rich blood. It's a symptom of coronary artery disease, the most common type of heart disease. One day while we were out shopping, my mother had a particularly scary angina attack. She was in her late-forties at the time and I was about 24. As we stopped at a traffic light on the way home, she turned to me, her face pale, her forehead damp with sweat, and said, "Bad hearts run in our family." Then she added, "You'll probably get angina, too."

I was struck by her tone of inevitability. The women in our family were predisposed to heart disease. Therefore hardening arteries and the possibility of untimely death must be my fate. Having witnessed the way in which my mother's life was curtailed by chronic sickness, by pain and fearfulness, I made a decision right there and then. Before the traffic light changed to green, I swore to myself, "I refuse to get angina. I reject my inheritance of heart disease."

Then I forgot all about it—at least, on a conscious level. I kept up with exercise, not out of any dedicated health promotion plan, but just because I enjoyed the feeling I got after running or going to the gym—the oxygen fizzing in my blood, the mental clarity, and the sensation of being limber. Exercise, and my work based in a large public health organization, also reminded me on a regular basis how incredible the human body is. Its capacity for repair is immense.

On turning 50, I found myself in good health, but I signed up for a complete physical check anyway. After the cardio workup, attached to electrodes, running on a treadmill that gradually sloped uphill, the technician told me that my stats were those of a person at least ten years younger than my biological age, and I suddenly remembered that long-ago moment in the car with my mother. I really hadn't thought about it in all those intervening years, but now I realized that I had passed through my forties without even a hint of angina. No chest pains. No high cholesterol. No angioplasty. No early grave. My heart was in good shape and I had altered my medical destiny.

Looking back, I believe I owe my fundamentally good health and my productiveness to a lifelong habit of exercise.

Not all of that exercise was super-intense. For long periods, especially when I was busy with a growing family and a full-time job, my routine consisted of brisk walking—but walking regularly maintained my baseline fitness, so that when I swung back into more challenging forms of exercise, it didn't take long to get up to speed.

Exercise has made a positive difference in my life. I exercised my way out of antenatal depression twice, and was able to deal with accidental injury and get through some stressful moments without collapsing. Now I am enjoying not only the benefits of exercise, but being able to keep up with my kids. Believe me, going for a hike with a fit 20-year-old calls for stamina.

Exercise is brilliant. It's the best and simplest way to insure ourselves against the onset of debilitating, chronic ill-health and it's also a straightforward, cost-effective way of managing existing health conditions. Better still, you can use exercise to target specific health conditions, such as arthritis, diabetes, stress, or irritable bowel syndrome. Even people with conditions such as fibromyalgia or epilepsy, who were once considered too vulnerable for exercise, have been shown in the latest health-care studies to benefit from cautious physical activity.

What this book does

Body Moves examines more than 50 common health conditions and describes how specific exercises can help to reduce their symptoms and stave off illness. It explains why exercise benefits these conditions, which kinds of exercise are best for specific infirmities, and how often you need to exercise to make a positive difference to them. *Body Moves* also offers best-exercise suggestions for life's normal experiences, such as menstruation, pregnancy, and aging.

Some recommendations are aerobic, or muscle-strengthening, while others focus on flexibility, stretching, and balance. Variety is important. Everyone gets bored eventually, doing the same thing over and over. If the shine wears off your aerobics classes at the gym, try salsa dancing for a change, if that is appropriate for your health status, or aqua aerobics. If you've always dismissed yoga because it's too "soft," try ashtanga or power yoga. Discover the conviviality of team sports or the mind-body pleasures of low-impact, non-contact martial arts. There's nothing more life-enhancing than a flexible mind in a flexible body.

In addition to researching the literature regarding exercise recommendations for common chronic conditions, I also found that online discussion groups were invaluable for hearing "from the horse's mouth," as it were, which exercise works for people with a particular ailment and which does not. For example, if I read that yoga was beneficial for a person with essential tremor, I then went to view the essential tremor online forum to see what people with ET actually had to say about their experiences with yoga and other forms of exercise.

A directory at the back of *Body Moves* lists the physical disciplines recommended throughout the book and offers descriptions of them and their variants. If you are new to exercise, please seek advice from your doctor and then from an instructor in the appropriate activity. When you begin a new exercise regime with an instructor, always inform him or her if you have a condition, disease, or impairment that may place limits on your physical ability, so that he or she knows to find ways to keep you safe.

Move your body and change your life

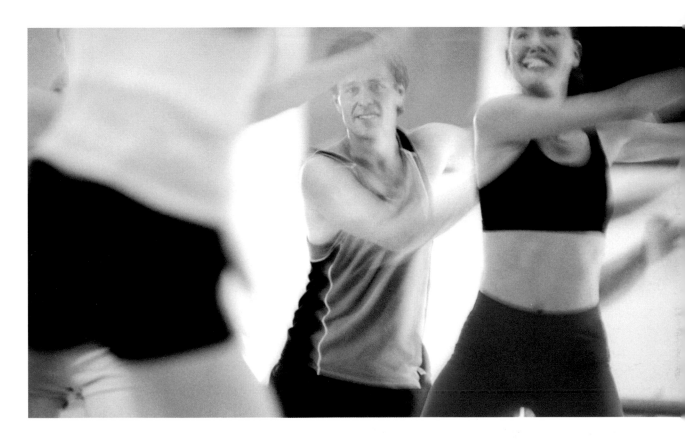

Some people would rather lose weight by starving themselves than burn fat through aerobic activity. "Exercise is so boring," they say. "I can't be bothered." Others would rather deal with stress by exercising their drinking arm, or give their thumbs a workout on a remote control device, than head out for a run or a swim. "I need to unwind," they say, "and with a workload like mine, I've got no time for exercise."

It's true that dedicated physical activity does take time and effort, two expenditures already

Challenge your preconceptions. Search for new ways to be active rather than getting bored and quitting.

under pressure in our demanding, overscheduled lives. It's normal to find exercise a little tedious after the first flush of enthusiasm passes and we make the transition from the beginner phase of a program to the reality of sustaining the exercise long term. (What?! You expect me to abandon this snuggly, toasty bed to go out and run in the rain? Are you kidding?!)

There can hardly be a person alive who doesn't know that hauling your butt off that couch can help prevent chronic disease, manage infirmities, and almost certainly prolong your life, but we wouldn't be human if we didn't ignore sound advice. Four out of ten cases of breast cancer in the United Kingdom could be prevented right now if women eased up on alcohol consumption, lost some weight, and got involved in regular exercise. It's that simple. But probably three out of those four women would rather take the risk of contracting cancer than make the effort to pull on a pair of sneakers and get started on a walking program. These are not bad women. These are human women. It's in our natures to be contrary, to say, "Yeah, cigarettes are harmful," while smoking a cigarette.

Our brains love to trick us into thinking that Buying The Thing (new running shoes, tennis racket, workout clothes) and Talking About The Thing ("They say yoga's brilliant!" "One day powerwalking will change my life!" "In the future, I intend to swim!" blah-blah-blah) are the same as Doing The Thing. They are not.

The point about physical activity is that you have to do it. It doesn't work to say, "I own a rebounder therefore I rebound."

But once you embark on exercise, you will find that exercise becomes its own best advocate for continuing to work out, even when you have one of those slumpy days when you don't particularly feel like doing it. It takes about 12 weeks of regular physical activity to wire the doing of it into your body's cellular memory. After that, your body gets used to moving around in a meaningful way. In fact, your muscles come to expect the swim or the bike ride, the run or the tai chi class. You certainly notice the difference in how you feel when you miss your regular session. When you can't exercise, you feel less energetic and life seems to be a little more uphill than it was the day before.

It can be frustrating when you begin on a new course of exercise and have to confront your limitations and your issues with self-belief and self-image, fear and negative thinking. But sometimes you need to move out of your comfort zone (as long as you are not pushing yourself too hard and risking injury or fatigue) to achieve the quality of life that you deserve. Committing to exercise as a sustained relationship with life requires the same kind of big-picture thinking and one-day-at-a-time actions as any other significant long-term undertaking, such as marriage, professional development, or bringing up children. The experience will have its ups and downs, joys and doubts, difficulties and breakthroughs, but when you stick with it, your sincere effort will be rewarded. It is absolutely worth the investment of time and energy. The payoff is that you will transform and preserve your life.

Sooner or later your body will send you a message

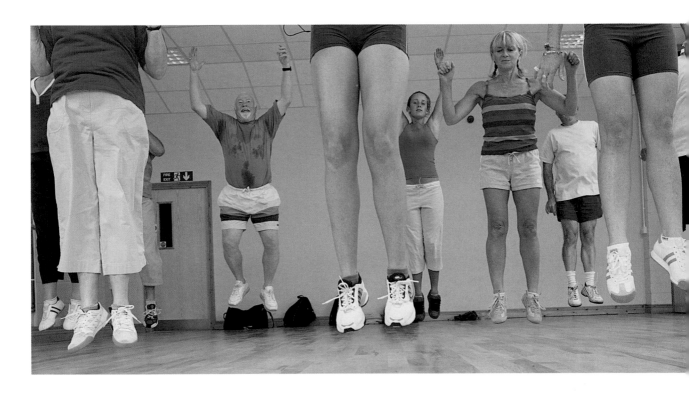

One Christmas morning a few years ago, a 46-year-old friend of mine was lying in bed with a hangover, after a staff party, trying to gather all of his mental and physical resources to get out of bed. He's a good person who loves his family and is a conscientious provider, but the demands of running his own business had got out of control. Business trips, entertaining clients, and long hours in his workshop had taken their toll on his health and his marriage. He had hardly seen anything of his kids for the whole of December, but he had promised that he would take time off over the holidays to be with his family.

Exercise patience. The benefits of physical activity tend to arrive in the form of a slow-release reward rather than a lottery-winning bonanza.

So he made the effort to roll out of bed and something cataclysmic happened to his spine. He fell onto the floor in excruciating pain from a slipped disk pressing on nerve roots and causing paralysis of some muscles. He lay there for the next hour unable to move, his calls for help unheard as the preparations for Christmas dinner went on downstairs without him. Eventually, one of his children found him, an ambulance was

11

called, and he was stretchered out, past the festive table and his anxious family, in the worst physical and emotional torment he had ever felt.

He spent the holidays in bed, doped up on painkillers, waiting for physical therapy. That was his wake-up call. His stint in rehabilitation reacquainted him with the therapeutic power of exercise and helped him to heal not only his back but also his injurious lifestyle.

"The thing that drove me crazy while I was in hospital," he says, "is that this was totally avoidable. I had wrecked myself."

Often we have to listen to the message many times before we act on it, but there's nothing like the shock of illness, trauma, or a devastating diagnosis to make us finally pledge to recover our health. Three factors are needed to promote health, as well as recovery following a significant illness: physical activity, mental stimulation, and social involvement.

Anyone who has experienced the pain, distress, and sheer inconvenience of illness and functional disability understands the value of health and wellbeing. It is more important than material possessions, status, and reputation. The only condition that enhances our lives more is love. When you love someone—your spouse, your partner, your children, your parents, your friends—you have everything to live for. That's a compelling reason to take care of your health.

Obesity and lack of exercise are the prime causes of many common diseases.

Type 2 diabetes—which leads to heart disease, vascular problems, high blood pressure, kidney failure, and weight-dependent arthritis—is at epidemic proportions around the world. The costs and impact of obesity, for both individuals and health services, are enormous. In the United States three out of four adults will be overweight by 2015 and 41 percent of the population will be obese. Almost two-thirds of British adults and a third of children are either overweight or obese. It is estimated that by 2015, health complications arising from obesity will cost the United Kingdom's National Health Service £6.3 billion. Nearly 18 percent of Australians are grossly overweight. In fact, the air ambulances that fly Australians from remote areas to city hospitals have had to be refitted to accommodate increasingly supersized patients.

Along with obesity, lack of exercise, and a rubbishy diet, prolonged stress has an insidious effect on health. Organs constantly flooded with stress hormones that raise blood pressure and heart rate, and constrict intestines, are likely to develop chronic disease. The immune system is affected. Depression may follow, or agitation that makes you a misery to yourself and others. Participating in regular exercise gives you a sense of control and of purpose, which is the key to reducing stress.

What getting physical will do for you

CURB CHRONIC DISEASE

Most chronic diseases arise from harmful lifestyle choices and are preventable. Whatever your age, gender, physical ability, or circumstances, if it's possible for you to move some part of your body somehow, you can use regular exercise to change your life for the better and keep at bay the most prevalent chronic health conditions that lead to premature death and disability: heart disease, high blood pressure, stroke, pulmonary conditions, arthritis, type 2 diabetes, osteoporosis, certain kinds of cancer, and mental illness.

BANISH BAD HABITS

Once you get into the good habit of exercising, it's much easier to let go of the bad habits in your life. Smoking and excessive alcohol consumption just don't mix with aerobic exercise. Taking care of yourself through exercise makes you more inclined to look after yourself in other ways too, by eating less and sleeping better.

MANAGE SOFT-TISSUE INJURY

Accidents will happen—although you might find that practicing a mind/body discipline, such as yoga, tai chi, or qigong, will teach you to be more aware and avoid crashes, collisions, and falls. Even after a muscle has healed, the area may remain weak and unstable, and the muscle tightened by scar tissue. Gentle exercise will encourage muscle strength, increase range of motion, and stabilize joints. Yoga is effective for

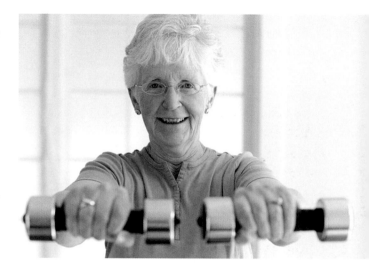

Regular exercise combined with a healthy diet can reduce the risk of developing Alzheimer's disease by as much as 60 percent.

soft-tissue injuries because it stretches tight muscles and promotes physical and mental relaxation, helping to disperse post-injury tension. Pilates is also a beneficial therapy for back or neck pain and healthy spine maintenance.

CONTROL YOUR WEIGHT

You've got just one body, so don't overload it or it will seize up and bog down way ahead of time. Dropping those extra pounds is the key to living longer and avoiding a raft of chronic diseases. To lose weight, you need to burn calories. Exercise burns calories. You can start exercising right now by putting one foot in front of the other and

13

walking out your door. Walk around the block. That's how easy it is. Do the same thing again tomorrow. Take the stairs instead of the elevator. Put on some music and dance. Increasing your physical activity by just five minutes each day will banish lethargy and give you the confidence to do more until you feel ready to commit to a dedicated fat-burning program.

INCREASE YOUR ENERGY

When your cardiovascular system is clogged and pressured, you lack pep, zing, and general *joie de vivre*. You find it hard to get your breath walking uphill or up a flight of stairs and everything feels like a drag, an effort. Once you get involved in aerobic exercise, you will notice the difference right away. Your blood starts pumping oxygen and nutrients into your tissues and your heart and lungs work more efficiently, making you feel invigorated and alive. Regular exercise helps keep high blood pressure under control. It lowers "bad" cholesterol, the kind that builds up plaque on the walls of your arteries, and increases "good" cholesterol. Your blood flows smoothly through your arteries, delivering yet more oxygen and nutrients, expanding your capacity for more exercise, and enhancing your feeling of vitality.

Opposite: *Physical workouts reduce tension by stimulating the production of endorphins—anti-stress chemicals—in the brain.*

IMPROVE YOUR MOOD

There's a reason why, when you are strung out and stressed, you keep doing the very things that make you strung out and stressed, even though you know you are stuck in a horrible rut. Sustained stress actually alters your neural circuitry. The parts of the brain that initiate decision-making and goal-seeking behavior atrophy, while those associated with repetition and compulsiveness expand. Fortunately, the brain is an adaptable organ and it has been proved that relaxation and exercise act as a circuit breaker. New studies have also found that regular physical activity can trigger a process that repairs the shriveled synaptic connections in your brain, allowing you to make decisions and feel in control of your life, while at the same time reducing the areas of neural cells that are responsible for the same old routine behavior. You start to feel happier and more relaxed. That in turn gives you confidence and improves self-esteem.

SLOW THE EFFECTS OF AGING

Poor health does not have to be an inevitable consequence of aging. A new study from the Stanford University School of Medicine, which tracked 500 older runners for more than two decades, found that aerobic exercise is associated with a longer life. Elderly joggers have fewer disabilities, remain fit for longer than non-runners, and are half as likely to die early deaths. Judicious use of the low-impact activities provided by elliptical trainers, spin classes, and swimming enables older people to maintain aerobic training far into later life. Resistance and strength training will also halt the slide into decrepitude. Even a small increase in muscle tone, through strength and balance exercises, can make a big difference in a frail person's ability to avoid falls and their injury-related hospitalizations. Walking, yoga, tai chi, and light weight training are all excellent ways to maintain fitness and flexibility.

KEEP YOUR THINKING SHARP

Cognitive decline used to be considered an inevitable result of getting older. While your brain's acuity does reduce from its peak of efficiency in your twenties, researchers are finding that a drop-off in cognitive performance can be forestalled by physical, as well as mental, exercise. Even moderate levels of physical activity, such as walking, can limit declines in cognition, but the real key to toning your circulatory system is more strenuous aerobic exercise, such as running, hiking, racket sports, swimming, cycling, and aerobic dance. Physical activity has been shown specifically to bolster memory and reduce the risk of dementia.

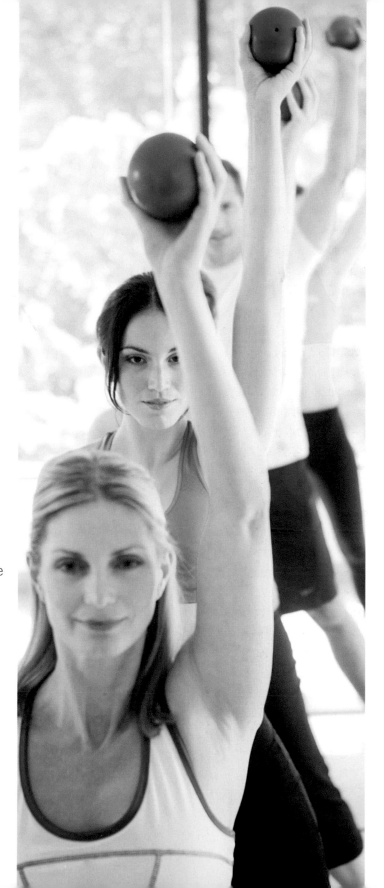

Wheelchair exercise

Exercise is good for everyone, including people with high levels of disability. If you are confined to a wheelchair for long hours, you will absolutely benefit from a fitness program that gets you moving your body as much as possible. Regular wheelchair exercise will increase your strength and flexibility, improve your mobility, strengthen your heart and lungs, and also help you to control your weight.

An exercise regime presents a challenge if you have limited movement. Many gyms are inadequate when it comes to accommodating people with disabilities safely, but facilities do exist for exercisers in wheelchairs. Do some online research to find what is available near you. Otherwise, you can work out at home to DVDs specifically designed for people in wheelchairs.

If you are the competitive type, look for an organized sport that you could play, such as wheelchair basketball, tennis, rugby, or racing. A social workout, such as wheelchair dancing, might suit you. Try wheelchair versions of the holistic exercises yoga and tai chi. A study at the University of Tennessee found that a simple seated tai chi program for people with an ambulatory disability greatly improved upper-body mobility and improved stamina and emotional wellbeing.

It's never too late to start

Getting in touch with your dynamic self, even if all you do is rotate your wrists or reach one arm in the air, will change your life for the better. Guaranteed. Don't neglect your body. It can help you to avoid years of chronic pain and internal disorders, and even if you are confined to a wheelchair, once your body gets used to its daily fix of oxygen, energy, and calming endorphins, there's no turning back. You will be better for it in every way. Pain and impairment is a state that restricts you mentally as well as physically. When people heal, they turn outward again, become less preoccupied by self and more sympathetic to the welfare of others.

A person's beliefs about his or her illness or impairment can significantly affect its outcome. Physical activity can foster hope and belief that improvement in your health status is possible. Find inspiration in the countless stories in print and online that document the ways in which people have managed disease and ailments, and encouraged injuries to heal, through dedicated physical activity. In almost every case, they have discovered along the way that a valuable internal transformation has taken place as well, resulting in a more integrated, better balanced, and happier person.

Chapter 1

Getting Started

You don't have to turn into a fitness maniac. The amount and level of exercise you do is as important as the type, and even small amounts produce improvements in health. Just 30 minutes of moderate walking five times a week can boost energy and help you lose some weight. But if you seriously want to burn fat and maintain an optimal cardiovascular system, you will need to up the level of aerobic intensity in your exercise routine.

A classic fitness program ideally combines aerobic and anaerobic exercises with activities that develop flexibility, coordination, and balance. Paying attention to mindful relaxation and stress reduction is also increasingly being seen as important in a balanced program.

Let's look at what balanced exercise involves in its most general sense. The recommendations for frequency and intensity of exercise given in this book naturally vary according to the condition being addressed, but a person without very limiting impairments could expect to follow the guidelines below.

Aerobic exercise

Aerobic means "with oxygen." This is endurance exercise using large muscle groups and is done at a pace that allows an adequate supply of oxygen to reach your muscles as you work out.
Examples: Walking, running, cycling, skiing, skating, dancing, swimming, hiking, rowing, using aerobic exercise machines.

Benefits: Trains the heart, lungs, and cardiovascular system to deliver oxygen more quickly and efficiently to every part of the body. As your heart grows stronger, you gain the capacity to work out more vigorously and for longer, and to recover more quickly from exercise. Aerobic activity burns fat tissue.
How often? Between three and five times per week.
How hard? You should work out at 55–80 percent of your maximum heart rate. Known as the target heart-rate zone, this is considered to be the best range for improving aerobic fitness. Beginners should work at the low end of the range and increase intensity as appropriate. You can easily find your maximum heart rate, measured in beats per minute (bpm), by subtracting your age from 220. Then find your target zone by working out the percentages. When you use aerobics machines at a gym, such as a stationary bike, treadmill, or rowing machine, you may be able to track your heart rate using the monitor on the machine.
Duration: People with low levels of fitness should maintain a heart rate of around 60 percent for a minimum of 15 minutes, not including warming up and cooling down. Those with a greater degree of fitness can exercise for 20 to 60 minutes in their target heart-rate zone.

Anaerobic exercise

Anaerobic exercise, meaning "without oxygen," involves rapid, brief bursts of strenuous activity in which you push your muscles to the limits in order to promote the growth of muscle tissue. Anaerobic exercise is short and intense, because oxygen is not used for energy. A by-product, lactic acid, contributes to muscle fatigue and must be burned up by the body during a recovery period before another anaerobic bout of exercise can take place.

Examples: Weight lifting (strength training), sprinting, jumping, sit-ups, push-ups, chin-ups, and squats. Strength or resistance training of muscles usually involves compound exercises and isolation exercises. Compound exercises, which use more than one muscle group, are the most effective for losing weight. Examples include bench press, push-ups, squats, shoulder press, and deadlifts. Isolation exercises use one muscle group and include bicep curls, tricep extensions, and leg extensions.

Benefits: Develops muscle mass, strength, and power. The more muscle you have, the more calories you are able to burn.

How often? Use resistance machines and weights to exercise each part of the body once or twice per week. You can exercise different muscles on different days (referred to as split routines) or train your whole body at each workout.

How hard? For those new to resistance training, compound exercises are best. Once you have a basic level of strength, you can add isolation exercises to your workouts for variety and to help shape individual muscles. Choose a weight that challenges you, but does not strain you to lift up

to 15 times in succession (referred to as a set). When you can perform more than 15 repetitions without rest, increase the weight slightly for your next workout. If you are training your whole body each time you exercise, do one or two exercises for each muscle group and perform up to three sets of each one. If you are doing a split routine, limit yourself to two or three exercises per muscle group and two or three sets of each exercise.

Duration: Beginners should exercise from 20 to 40 minutes, resting between sets for two or three minutes. Work up to 60 minutes as you become fitter, resting for a minute or less between sets.

Skill development exercise

Skill development includes flexibility, balance, rhythm, and coordination.

Examples: Tennis, golf, exercises with Swiss balls, resistance bands, and wobble boards, and stretching with breath control and meditation (yoga, tai chi, and Pilates).

Benefits: Muscular coordination, flexibility, balance, and tone. Balance, rhythm, and coordination challenges help to integrate the function of left and right brain hemispheres, stimulate the muscles and nervous system, and help prevent injury. Psychological benefits include a reduction in stress and promotion of a greater sense of wellbeing.

How often? Between three and five times a week.

Duration: Up to 60 minutes per session taking rest as required.

Easing into exercise

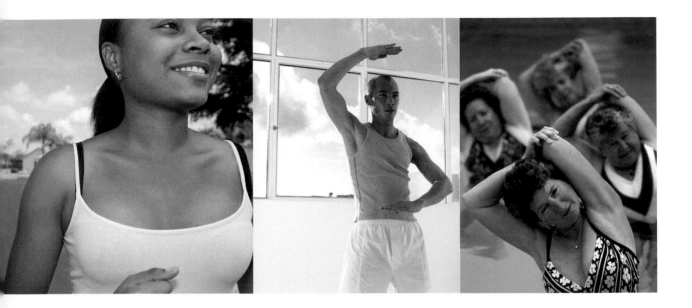

Start simple

Don't embark on an overly ambitious routine that
will exhaust you after the first couple of outings,
especially if you've been sedentary for a long time.
If you are a stranger to physical activity, you need
to go through a conditioning period of around six
weeks of consistent workouts to get in good
enough shape for exercise to feel comfortable.

Begin by walking for 15 minutes per day, or try
gentle aqua aerobics. Add a qigong class to
familiarize yourself with forgiving balance and
body movements, or a gentle yoga class to get
used to stretching. Older and novice exercisers
should always factor in plenty of recovery time.

*Warm up first for at least five minutes, so that your heart
is pumping more oxygenated blood to your muscles.*

Listen to your body

Forget the old adage of "No pain, no gain." If any
part of you is hurting, pay attention and seek
advice. Don't compare your performance with
others. You are exercising enough if you break
out into a light sweat, but are still capable of
talking. When exercising, you should always be in
an aerobic state, which means that you have
enough oxygen in your blood to be able to hold a
conversation. If you find yourself gasping and
unable to speak, then slow down and take it easy.

Five effective aerobic workouts for good health

Running

This is the most popular cardio workout around. All you need is a good pair of running shoes, a pair of shorts, a T-shirt, and you're away. Running burns calories and builds aerobic capacity.

Warm up: Walk for five minutes, then walk and jog slowly for up to ten minutes before easing into your running pace. Cool down by reversing this procedure.

Pace yourself: Start by running easily achievable distances and gradually increase speed and distance on successive weeks.

Rest: If you are feeling fatigued (as opposed to feeling lazy), take a day off.

Power walking

Convenient and accessible, power walking can be done by anyone, including older people. These fast-walking sessions will build endurance, burn fat, and increase your heart rate. Like running, all you require are good training shoes and comfortable clothing to get started.

Warm up: Walk at an easy pace for five to ten minutes. Then stop and slowly do flexibility and stretching exercises for five minutes.

Pace yourself: Continue at a pace that brings your heart rate up to 70 percent of your maximum.

Swimming

An excellent low-impact workout, swimming increases lung capacity and tones the body. You will need swimming goggles, a cap, a swimsuit, and access to a pool. Swim fins, leg floats, and kickboards are optional.

Warm up: Swim 250–400 meters, using freestyle, backstroke, and breaststroke.

Pace yourself: Do 2x50-meter drills, such as two kicks to one pull in breaststroke; scissors kick while extending the arms in front, turning the head to the side to breathe; scissors kick on the right side while extending the right arm only, repeated on the left side. Pause every 25 meters. Finish the workout by doing 2x100 meters each of backstroke and breaststroke, and 10x50 meters

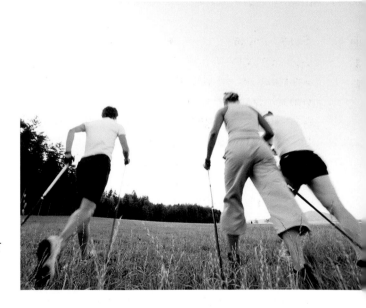

Don't think about speed when you first start power walking. Concentrate on finding a stride that feels comfortable, even if it's just a shuffle.

of freestyle. Rest for 60 seconds. Cool down by doing 150 meters of easy strokes, and then some stretches when you get out of the pool.

Boxing

An intense cardio workout, boxing burns calories ferociously, builds strength, and tones the body. You can sign up for one-on-one sessions with a boxing instructor or attend boxfit classes at a gym, where you will join a group following a 45 to 60 minute routine led by an instructor. Boxing gloves are provided at boxfit gym classes, but you will need to bring your own cotton inners. Condition the body for boxing by first establishing a consistent running routine. Boxfit classes combine resistance endurance training, including running and machine work, with boxing drills that use multiple punches and defensive techniques. You will also do timed rounds, punching light to heavy bags.

Ashtanga yoga

Ashtanga is a form of yoga that involves continuous movement. Its postures are linked with jumps, and synchronized with the breath. The aim is to purify the body by sweating out toxins. It is also a total cardio workout for every part of the body and builds core strength and flexibility. You will need to attend classes at first to be taught the correct sequence of postures and techniques for achieving them, but after that you can practice on your own. You will need a yoga mat and workout clothes. The ashtanga primary series arranges the postures in sequence for optimal performance beginning with a warm-up of sun salutations, proceeding through standing and sitting postures, inversions, and relaxation. The cardiovascular benefits of ashtanga quickly become apparent if it is practiced three to six times a week.

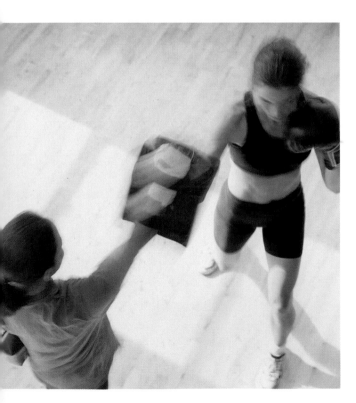

Boxing training develops agility, endurance, speed, and power, and is a great aerobic workout. Taking up boxing training is a good way to achieve a high level of fitness.

Motivation

If you are struggling with motivation, despite everything you know about how much you need this exercise and how good it will be for you, you are not alone. Even the most advanced runners say that getting your shoes on is the hardest part of any workout.

The well-known fitness enthusiast and adventurer Sir Ranulph Fiennes, who climbed Mount Everest in 2009 at the age of 65, has an effective tactic for bamboozling the voice in your head that is making excuses for not working out. He says you should simply stand up at once. This interrupts the flow of negative thoughts and is in itself a physical action. If you are already standing up, you should stop what you are doing and head for your exercise shoes and clothes without another thought. If you plan to exercise in the morning, lay out your clothes the night before, so that you can put them on as soon as your alarm goes off without thinking about it. Do it automatically and don't give a thought to the exercise session you are about to embark on. Walk out the door.

Have fun: Do everything you can think of to make exercising a pleasure. If you like dressing up in fancy workout clothes, go for it! Once you've bought it all, you don't want to waste it, right? You are more likely to make room for regular exercise if you transform your perception of it from being a task to an occasion to socialize, and to nurture yourself.

Book it and log it: Make exercise appointments with yourself. Write them in your diary and on your calendar so that your exercise times become embedded into your daily or weekly routine.

As well as that, keep a log book or journal of the days you exercised—what you did and how you felt. Reading back over your progress will encourage you.

People power: Recruit an exercise buddy. It's often easier to stick to your exercise routine when you have to stay committed to a friend, partner, or colleague. You could also involve yourself in group exercise—dancing, for example, or tennis. The incentives to turn up and play or dance are much greater when teammates and friends are involved.

Distract yourself: Play music or download audiobooks or podcasts to listen to while you work out. Upbeat music primes the body systems needed for high-energy movement, but listening to anything you enjoy makes the session fun and can often boost your performance.

Embrace variety: Mix it up. Try a range of classes at the gym and different types of yoga, or set yourself a new walking or running route.

Incentivize yourself: Stop each session at the point where you think you can do more. You will be eager to get back to it.

Check with your doctor

Although physical activity is perfectly safe for most people, it is wise to consult your doctor before you start an exercise program. Mayo Clinic, the distinguished American medical practice, says that it is particularly important to seek advice from your doctor about a regimen of exercise if you have a medical condition, and if any of the following apply to you:

- You've had a heart attack.
- You have asthma or lung disease.
- You have diabetes or heart, liver, or kidney disease.
- You feel pain in your chest, joints, or muscles during physical activity.
- You have arthritis or osteoporosis.
- You've had joint replacement surgery.
- You experience symptoms such as loss of balance, dizziness, or loss of consciousness.
- You take medication to manage a chronic condition.
- You have an untreated joint or muscle injury, or persistent symptoms after a joint or muscle injury.
- You're pregnant.

The American College of Sports Medicine also recommends you see your doctor if two or more of the following apply:

- You're a man older than age 45 or a woman older than age 55.
- You have a family history of heart disease before age 55.
- You have high blood pressure or high cholesterol.
- You smoke or you quit smoking in the past six months.
- You're overweight or obese.

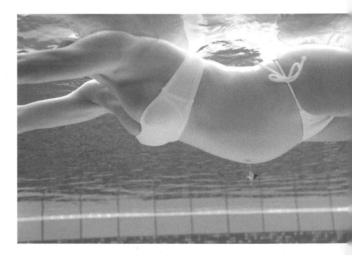

One of the safest ways to keep fit is to exercise in water and this is especially true if you are pregnant. Healthy women should be able to swim for the full nine months of their pregnancy. (See pages 186–9 for more information.)

Chapter 2

Heart and Circulation

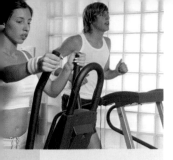

BEST MOVES

power walking

hiking

running

dancing

rope jumping

skating

cycling

skiing

aerobics classes

rowing

swimming

endurance sports

circuit training

Swimming and elliptical training are especially beneficial for people with knee problems.

Coronary artery disease

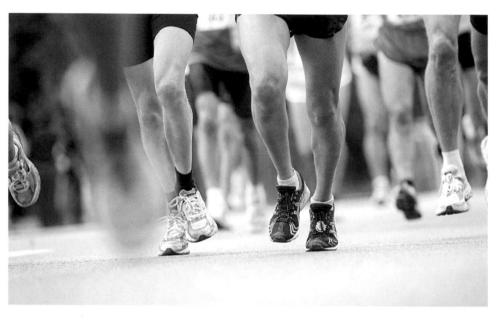

Cardiovascular disease accounts for the death of more people in the developed world than any other cause. Coronary artery disease is the most common manifestation of cardiovascular disease. It refers to the hardening and shrinking of the coronary arteries, a process called atherosclerosis, which diminishes blood flow and reduces oxygen supply to the heart muscle. This lack of oxygen may cause the chest pains of angina. If the coronary artery becomes completely blocked, a whole section of the heart muscle is deprived of oxygen and dies, resulting in a heart attack. Coronary artery disease is a progressive, silent disease that very often is unobserved until the first symptoms of heart attack occur.

Aerobic exercise, such as running, helps to prevent the development of coronary artery disease, as well as shifting excess weight and promoting better sleep.

Why exercise helps
Regular aerobic activity helps combat coronary artery disease because it delivers oxygen to the heart muscle, and improves lung function. It also increases stamina, burns excess fat, promotes sound sleep, and improves wellbeing.

Use your arms as well as your legs when you do aerobic exercise. Although peak heart rates are similar with arm and leg exercise, heart rate and blood pressure responses are higher during arm exercise than during leg exercise.

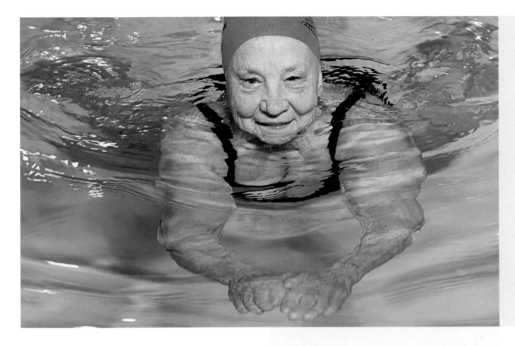

HOW OFTEN?
- At least 30 minutes of aerobic exercise daily.
- Try to include at least one swimming session per week.

However, note that dynamic arm movements may cause a rise in blood pressure in some people.

If the cardio machines in your gym are not equipped with heart-rate monitors, you can easily determine your heart rate by placing your index and middle fingers on your carotid artery (on the neck, to the side of the Adam's apple) or on your radial artery (wrist). Press firmly till you start feeling the throbbing sensation. Watch the timer on the cardio machine and count the heartbeats for 10 seconds. Multiply the result by 6. That's your heart rate.

Swimming tips
- Breathe out when your face is underwater and breathe in as soon as your face is out of the water. Your stroke will be smoother, faster, and more efficient.
- Try to use one breath for every three strokes.
- Use equipment, such as pull buoys and kickboards, to avoid unnecessary strain on the body.
- Mix up your workouts to incorporate endurance, technique, and speed. Do two stamina sessions followed by one speed session.

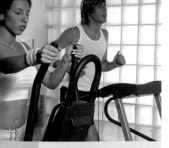

Coronary artery disease continued

Regular aerobic activity can help prevent the development of coronary artery disease.

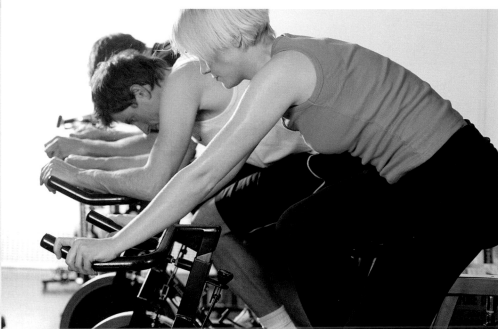

EXERCISE FOR PEOPLE WITH CORONARY ARTERY DISEASE

Although rest and palliative care have been traditionally prescribed for patients with heart failure, several recent studies have shown that physical exercise has a beneficial effect on people suffering from coronary artery disease or stable heart failure.

Exercise as a treatment is just as effective for older patients as for younger ones. A study presented at the 2009 congress of the European Association of Cardiovascular Prevention and Rehabilitation suggests that a moderate, supervised exercise program four times daily for four weeks can improve the function of the circulatory system. It improves arterial blood flow and helps to regenerate diseased tissue.

HOW OFTEN?

- **Warm up for five minutes with stretches followed by 10–20 minutes of cycling under supervision by a health professional on a stationary bicycle at 60–70 percent of maximal aerobic capacity. Cool down for five minutes.**

Stretches for swimmers

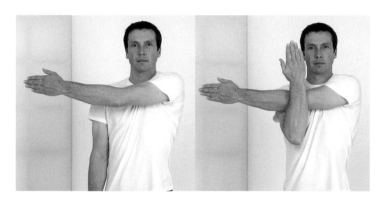

1. *Stretch your left arm across your chest. Bend your right arm over the left elbow and pull the left arm farther across your chest, keeping your left arm straight. Hold for 15 seconds and then repeat on the other side.*

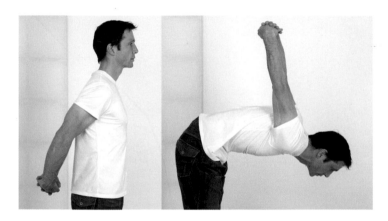

2. *Clasp your hands together behind your back. Bend forward and bring your hands over your head to stretch your shoulders and back.*

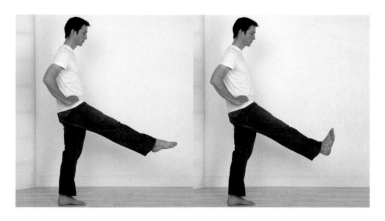

3. *Stand upright, hands on hips, and stretch one leg out in front of you. Point and flex your toes for a few seconds at a time. Repeat with the other leg.*

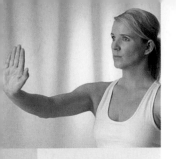

Angina

BEST MOVES

cycling on a stationary bike that has a heart-rate monitor and the capacity to set the pedal load and measure performance

walking on a treadmill that can monitor heart rate

qigong

tai chi

yoga

Angina is caused by narrowed coronary arteries that restrict the flow of blood to the heart muscle, increasing the risk of heart attack. A high cholesterol level and diabetes can also lead to angina. Stable angina occurs when a person feels acute pain or tightening in the chest during exertion, such as brisk walking or climbing stairs, or during an emotionally stressful event. Unstable angina is a more serious condition, where a person is gripped by chest pain during light physical exercise or sometimes even while resting.

Can exercise help angina?

People with angina should undertake an evaluation by a health professional in order to determine their responses to exercise. Generally, people with stable angina or with a high angina threshold measured at four METs or greater (MET means metabolic equivalent unit and measures oxygen uptake) should be able to undertake a supervised exercise program. If your angina threshold is two or three METS, exercise is probably not appropriate for you. If you experience greater than mild-to-moderate symptoms during an exercise session, you should stop exercising and consult a physician.

Why exercise helps

Although vigorous exercise may trigger angina, regular, moderate aerobic exercise, such as walking or qigong, can be an effective way of keeping angina in check, because it decreases heart rate and blood pressure.

Exercise also helps to disperse stress and encourages feelings of wellbeing and relaxation. It is important for people with angina to find ways of maintaining a calm emotional state. Stress, tension, and other forms of mental agitation can bring on an angina attack. Forms of exercise that have a gentle mind-body connection, such as yoga, qigong, and tai chi, are excellent activities for people who cannot tolerate stress on their hearts. Tai chi's calm, repetitive motions, for instance, work all of the major muscle groups of the body without raising the heart rate, and have a tranquil effect on the mind and the nervous system.

People with the kind of stable angina that responds well to physical activity may find that they can gradually exercise at higher intensities.

Opposite: *If you suffer from angina, see your doctor for advice before beginning an exercise program. Avoid vigorous workouts—walk rather than run on a treadmill.*

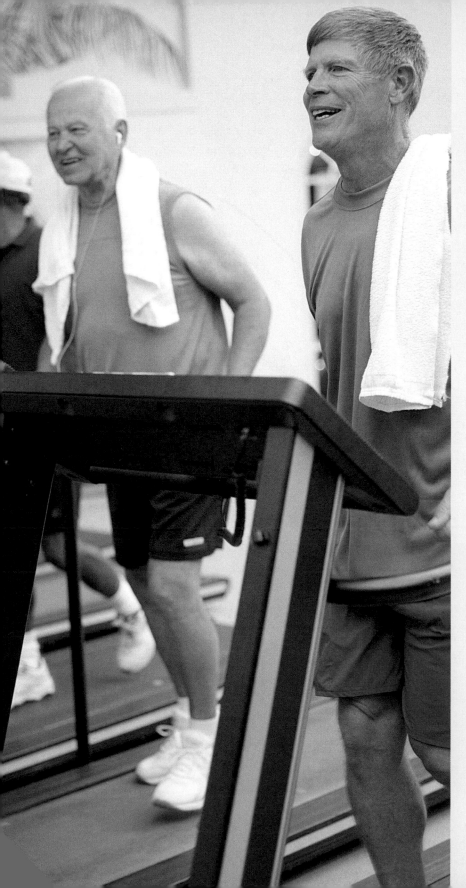

HOW OFTEN?

- Don't exercise alone if you have angina. If angina should occur during the session, stop exercising.
- Begin with a warm-up of at least 10 minutes of gentle stretches. Follow with an aerobic phase of 10–20 minutes at an intensity that is not greater than the warm-up. Alternate activity and rest until you have sufficient strength and endurance to sustain continuous exercise.
- Be aware of your breathing in order to minimize a tendency to hold the breath. The exercise cool-down period should be gradual and last at least 10 minutes.
- Try to attend at least one qigong, tai chi, or yoga class per week, and walk for around 10 minutes daily on a treadmill or outdoors.

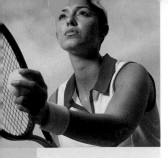

Stroke prevention

BEST MOVES

fast walking

jogging

running

cycling

dancing

swimming

aerobic gym classes

light weight lifting

racket sports

yoga

A stroke happens when a blood clot blocks an artery or vein, interrupting the flow of blood to an area of the brain, which damages those brain cells. You are likely to avoid having a stroke if you quit smoking, limit the amount of alcohol you drink, and stay at a healthy weight. Being overweight increases your risk of developing high blood pressure, high cholesterol, heart problems, and diabetes, all of which are risk factors for stroke.

Why exercise helps

Physical activity raises your heart rate and lowers your risk of stroke, partly by reducing the likelihood of incurring high blood pressure and heart disease, its two greatest risk factors. The more physically active you are, the lower your risk. Moderately active people have a 20 percent lower risk of stroke than inactive people. Highly active people have about a 30 percent reduction of risk. Research shows that people who are physically active before suffering a stroke may have less severe problems as a result, and recover better, compared with those people who did not exercise before having a stroke.

Opposite: *Fast walking on a regular basis can decrease the risk of stroke by 20 percent compared with people who don't exercise regularly.*

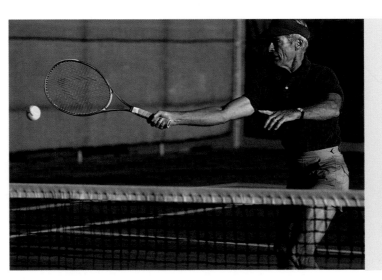

HOW OFTEN?
- **30 minutes per day, 5 days per week.**

Playing tennis and other racket sports can protect against stroke and help recovery.

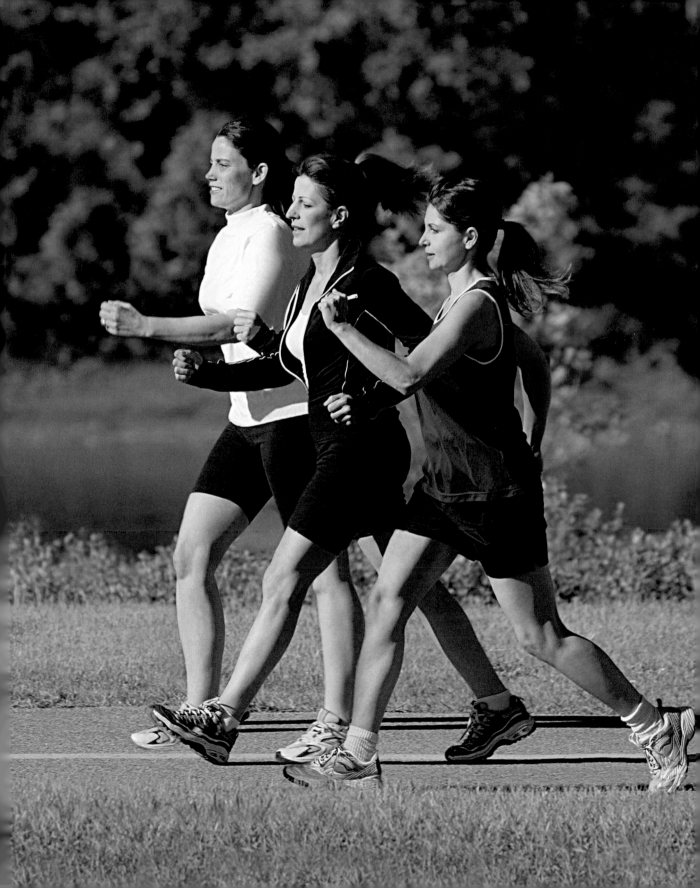

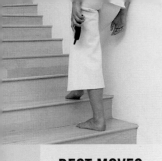

Peripheral arterial disease

Peripheral arterial disease (PAD) develops when the arteries that supply blood to the internal organs, arms, and legs become completely or partially blocked as a result of atherosclerosis. The impaired blood flow in the arteries often causes painful cramping of the leg muscles when walking.

Why exercise helps

Regular exercise encourages smaller arteries in the legs to enlarge, which improves blood supply. Exercise delays the onset of pain and increases mobility for people suffering with PAD. Walking has been shown to be the best exercise to improve symptoms. Your doctor may want you to try a supervised program, at first, with a physical therapist. Each day, you walk on a treadmill until your legs begin to hurt, rest, and then continue. The goal is to increase the amount of

time you can exercise before the pain starts. With your doctor's approval, you can embark on a similar walking program at home. After you can walk for 10 minutes without significant pain, add some stair climbing to your exercise routine. Use stairs instead of an elevator. As with walking, work out until pain becomes more than moderate, and increase the amount of stairs you climb as your legs improve.

If walking or stair climbing proves too difficult, you can increase aerobic fitness without using your legs, by means of an arm ergometer. This is a device similar to a stationary bike, but instead of rotating the pedal with the legs, handles are rotated with the arms. Other exercises, such as swimming and tai chi, will also help you to improve fitness, and are good for the heart, but these should be done in addition to walking.

Opposite: *A regular walking program with a friend will keep you motivated—and gradually decrease the pain of peripheral arterial disease.*

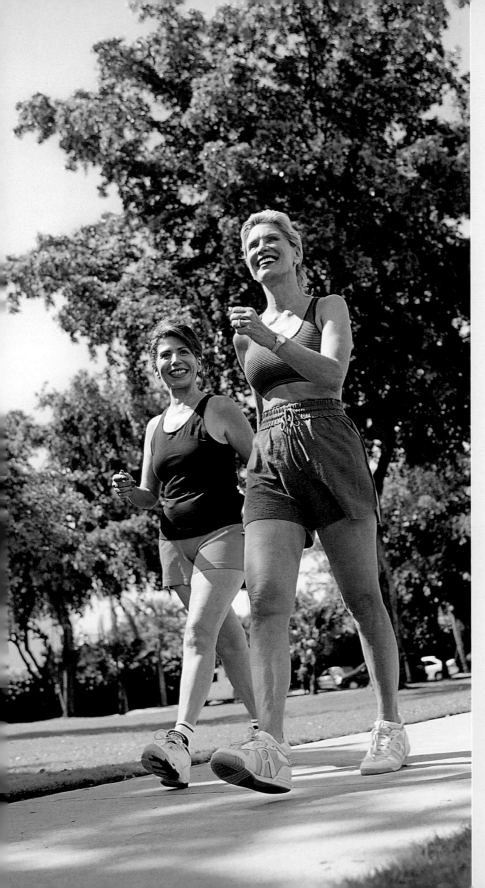

HOW OFTEN?

- Walking for 30 minutes 3 times per week can significantly improve endurance and slow the progression of peripheral arterial disease.
- Start by trying to walk for 6–8 minutes without stopping. You may experience pain, but unless the pain is too excruciating, try to tolerate it until you have completed 6 minutes. The pain is not damaging to the muscles.
- Rest for 5 minutes and then attempt another walk of 6–8 minutes. Continue until you have walked for 30 minutes.
- Walk at least 3 times per week. As the pain recedes, increase the amount of time that you walk before stopping. Eventually, walk every day, or on most days, preferably for up to an hour.

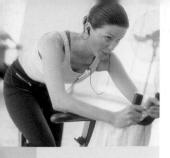

BEST MOVES

power walking

running

dancing

rope jumping

skating

cycling

skiing

aerobics classes

rowing

swimming

endurance sports

training on exercise machines

power yoga or ashtanga yoga

High cholesterol

Cholesterol is a fat (lipid) produced by the liver and is crucial for normal body functioning. It is transported in the blood by molecules called lipoproteins. Low-density lipoprotein (LDL) is often referred to as "bad" cholesterol. LDL carries cholesterol from the liver to cells, but if there is too much fat for the cells to use, the buildup of LDL can increase the risk of arterial disease (atherosclerosis or narrowed coronary arteries). High-density lipoprotein (HDL), known as "good" cholesterol, does the opposite of LDL. It prevents arterial disease by clearing cholesterol from the blood.

Why exercise helps

Regular exercise increases HDL, or good cholesterol, while decreasing LDL, or bad cholesterol, and minimizing the risk of developing coronary heart disease. Elevated levels of bad cholesterol are caused by a sedentary lifestyle, a diet high in saturated fats, and being overweight. Exercise can lower cholesterol by helping you to shed extra weight. It does this by stimulating enzymes that help move bad LDL from the blood to the liver, from where it can be excreted by the digestive system. The more you exercise, the more LDL your body expels.

Opposite: *Aerobic exercise, such as jumping rope, helps the body excrete LDL, or bad cholesterol, from the liver.*

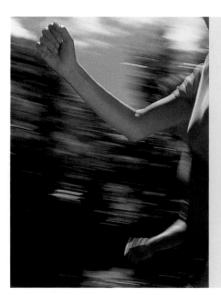

HOW OFTEN?

- A 2002 study by Duke University Medical Center in North Carolina found that it requires a good amount of exercise to lower cholesterol. Just walking is not enough.
- The American Heart Association recommends at least 60 minutes of high-intensity aerobic activity up to 5 times a week if you're trying to lose weight and lower cholesterol.
- You can get your exercise in 10- or 15-minute increments if need be, as long as it adds up to at least 60 minutes by the end of the day.

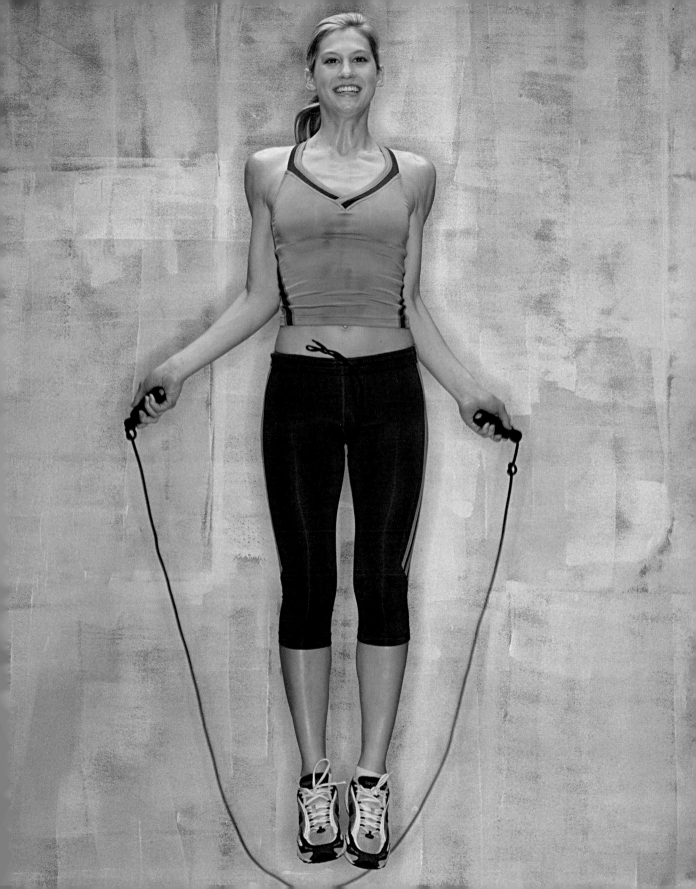

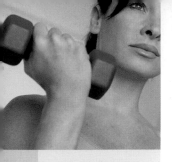

Varicose veins

BEST MOVES

swimming

walking

cycling

weight training

yoga

Around 30 percent of women develop enlarged, twisted veins, which look blue or purple, near the surface of the skin. They commonly appear on the legs and ankles, but can also affect the pelvis or uterus.

Arteries carry blood from the heart to your organs and tissues, while veins return the used blood to your heart, working against gravity. Veins become varicose when the tiny one-way valves that open to let the blood through and close to stop it going backward become weakened. When the valves don't function properly, blood can leak backward, collecting in the veins and causing them to enlarge. Risk factors for developing varicose veins are increasing age, pregnancy, being overweight, and a job that involves standing for long periods of time. Exercise can minimize the damage and ease the discomfort of varicose veins.

Why exercise helps

Varicose veins swell because blood pools in them. When you exercise, the pumping action of your leg muscles squeezes blood from the veins and directs it back toward the heart. Standing or sitting increases the pooling of blood in the veins.

Low-impact exercise is more therapeutic for varicose veins than high impact, because activities such as jogging or high-impact aerobics increase blood pressure in the legs, which weakens the veins. Moderate leg exercises help relieve varicose veins and reduce the aching associated with them.

Opposite: *Low-impact exercise, such as swimming, is good for varicose veins because it does not increase pressure in the veins.*

HEART AND CIRCULATION

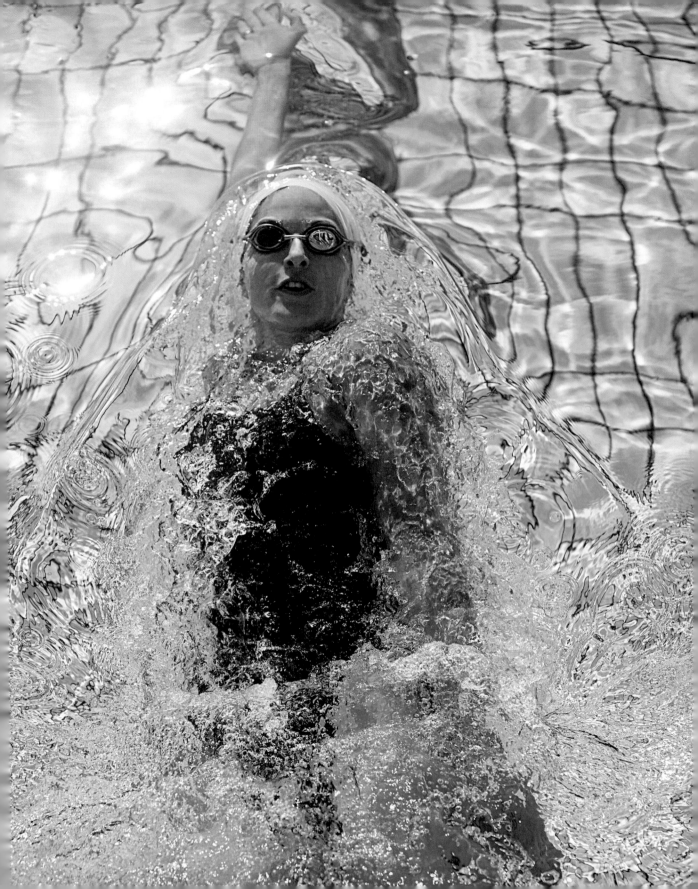

Leg exercises to improve blood flow

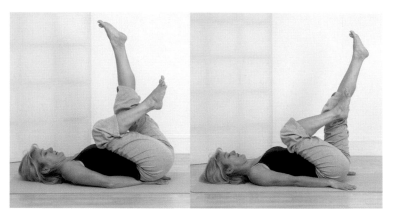

PEDALING

Lie on your back on the floor with your hands out to the side. If you feel some strain to the lower back, place your hands beneath your buttocks. Lift your legs off the floor and pedal them as if you were pedaling a bicycle. The more you elevate your legs, the more you will increase blood circulation to them. Continue this exercise for as long as you are comfortably able to do so.

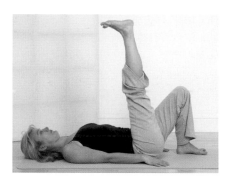

LEG LIFTS

Lie on your back, with your hands beneath your buttocks, if you wish. Keeping your buttocks pressed down, and your lower back against the floor, lift one leg at a time, keeping the other one bent with the foot flat on the floor. Hold the upright leg in an elevated position, perpendicular to the floor, until you feel the blood begin to flow back from your foot, calf, and thigh. Then repeat the exercise with your other leg. You could also lie with both legs up against a wall until you feel an improvement in blood circulation (see opposite).

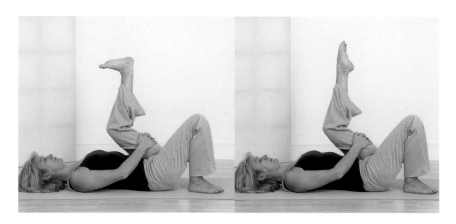

KNEE BENDS WITH ANKLE FLEXES

Lie on your back on the floor. Pull one knee in toward your chest by holding the leg behind the thigh. Keep the other leg bent, foot flat on the floor. Point and flex the foot of the raised leg several times. Do this attentively in order to exercise the calf muscles and the tendons around your ankle. Repeat with the other leg.

Yoga for varicose veins and tired legs

LEGS UP THE WALL AND SHOULDER STAND

These poses are ideal for improving circulation and strength in the legs, and promoting relaxation. In both, the legs are inverted and the pressure of gravity is reversed, reducing the pooled blood in the veins. Do these postures each day, holding them for 3–5 minutes. When you stand up, movement of fluids in the legs is greatly improved.

Follow these poses with the Corpse pose. Lie flat on your back with your feet hip-distance apart. Keep your head and spine in a straight line. This induces whole-body relaxation, placing the heart completely level with the rest of the body. Lie in this pose for as long as you like.

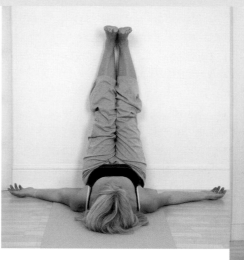

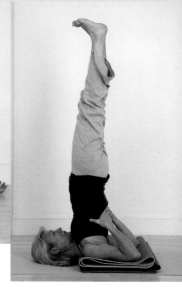

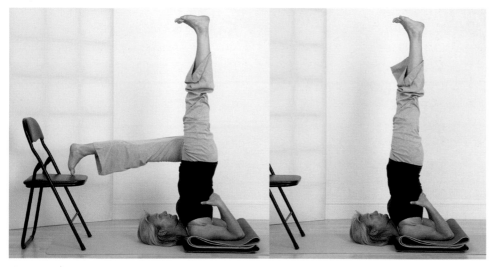

For instructions on how to get into these yoga positions, see page 73.

You can use a chair to help you achieve the Shoulder Stand position. Place a folded mat, small pillow, or rolled towel under your neck for comfort and support. People with a limited range of movement or high blood pressure should do the modified version of Shoulder Stand—either leave your feet on the chair or lie at a right-angle to the wall, lift your feet over your head, and place them flat on the wall.

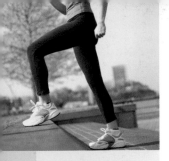

BEST MOVES

walking

running

cycling

swimming

rowing

dancing

yoga (except inversions)

tai chi

qigong

gardening

Blood pressure

The blood that runs through our veins and arteries, supplying oxygen to the body organs, is pumped in and out of the heart with a force that brings pressure to bear on the walls of the blood vessels. If this pressure increases, the heart has to pump harder to do its work and the arteries develop abnormal tissue growth, which decreases the flow of blood. As the heart works even harder to pump blood through narrowed arteries, the pressure on the arterial walls continues to increase. This high blood pressure (also known as hypertension) eventually weakens the heart. Stroke, heart attack, or kidney failure may be the result.

A blood pressure reading of 120/80 is considered normal in a healthy adult. If your blood pressure reaches 140/90 or higher on two separate occasions, you will be diagnosed with high blood pressure. The higher (systolic) number is a reading of the pressure in your blood vessels when your heart is beating at its maximum strength. The lower number (diastolic) tells you what the pressure is when your heart is at rest.

Why exercise helps

Losing weight and engaging in aerobic activity will strengthen your heart and so lower blood pressure—a stronger heart can pump more blood with less effort. Aerobic activities do it by increasing the body's oxygen consumption. The heart and circulatory system pump out more oxygenated blood to meet this increased need. If your blood pressure is normal, exercise can keep it from rising as you age. To maintain it, you need to keep exercising. It takes about one to three months of regular aerobic exercise to have an impact on your blood pressure, and the benefits last only as long as you continue to exercise. People with high blood pressure should avoid yoga inversions, such as Shoulder Stand and Headstand, since the cardiovascular changes caused by the body's being upside down are potentially damaging.

Everyday activities

Any moderate-level physical task that takes an effort and works large groups of muscles, such as your legs, arms, and shoulders, can help lower blood pressure. Plenty of everyday tasks as well as sporty activities involve useful aerobic effort:

- Climb stairs for 15 minutes
- Dance for 30 minutes
- Garden for 45 minutes
- Push a baby stroller 1½ miles in 30 minutes
- Rake leaves for 30 minutes
- Shovel snow for 30 minutes
- Wash and wax a car for 45 to 60 minutes
- Wash windows for 45 to 60 minutes

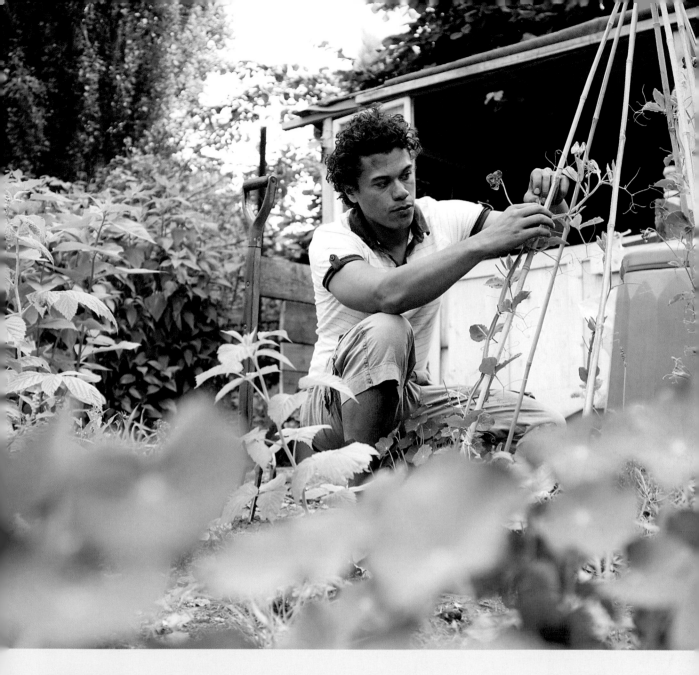

HOW OFTEN?

- At least 30 minutes of exercise per day will bring down blood pressure and improve circulation. Warm up by walking slowly or stretching for at least 10 minutes—longer for older people and those who have been sedentary for a long time. Then exercise for 30 minutes and cool down with 5 more minutes of light activity. Don't skimp on the cool-down. If you stop exercising too quickly, your blood pressure can drop sharply and cause painful muscle cramping.

Gardening for 45 minutes is a great way to help lower blood pressure.

>

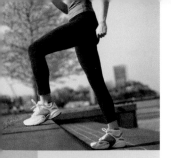

Blood pressure continued

If your blood pressure is normal, exercise can keep it from rising as you age.

Lifting weights

The sustained lifting required by bench-pressing heavy weights can be harmful if you have high blood pressure. Straining to hold a massive weight above your body forces your heart to pump blood into your arms at a rate that can raise blood pressure. If you want to add some weight training to your exercise program, choose repetitions of lighter free weights instead.

Similarly, be aware that strenuous arm exercises may cause a rise in blood pressure in some people, because heart rate and blood-pressure response during arm exercise are higher than they are during leg exercise.

Try something different

WALKING ON COBBLESTONES

Walk barefoot or in socks on cobblestones or on a manufactured cobblestone mat. Cobblestone walking has its roots in traditional Chinese medicine and it is common in China to see people walking on specially designed paths of river stones in large city parks as an exercise. Walking on specifically placed, uneven, natural stones stimulates the reflexes or acupressure points on the soles of the feet, which are linked to all organs and tissues of the body, and can produce health benefits. A study conducted at the Oregon Research Institute showed that walking on a cobblestone mat significantly reduced blood pressure and improved balance among adults of 60 years and older.

How often?
- **30 minutes each day.**

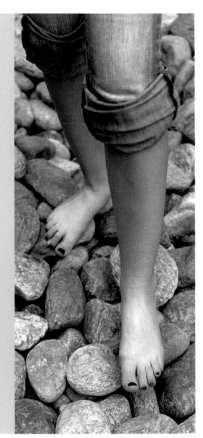

Chapter 3

Brain and Nervous System

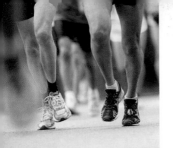

Epilepsy

BEST MOVES

walking

running

low-impact aerobics

yoga

qigong

tai chi

resistance and strength training with weights, machines, or a Swiss ball

Pilates

Epilepsy is caused by abnormal electrical activity within the brain, which results in seizures of varying severity. Some seizures affect part of the body only, or simply cause an alteration in the senses. Most people diagnosed with epilepsy take anti-seizure medications. Sound sleep, adequate nutrition, and physical activity are also encouraged. Some people with epilepsy avoid exercise because they are afraid it will bring on a seizure. In fact, it is rare for a person to have an epileptic seizure while exercising. With appropriate precautions, most people with epilepsy can participate in some type of exercise or sporting activity.

Why exercise helps

Physical conditioning boosts confidence and self-esteem as well as fitness. Research has shown that the improved fitness and wellbeing that come from exercising, and the relaxing practice of yoga, qigong, or tai chi, result in some people with epilepsy having fewer seizures. There are several reasons for this. The heavy breathing associated with exercise prevents carbon dioxide from building up in the blood. Regular exercise effectively calms the brain and helps to manage stress, a known seizure trigger. The concentration needed to exercise may focus the brain so that seizures are less likely.

Precautions

- Make sure that the people with whom you are exercising are aware of your condition and know what to do if you have a seizure.
- Let family or friends know your walking or jogging route before you leave and roughly how long you will be out.
- If you choose to participate in contact sports, such as football or hockey, wear a helmet and proper pads.
- Don't undertake water sports alone. Swim with companions who are aware of your condition, and who are physically strong enough to support you and know what to do if you have a seizure.
- Avoid scuba diving, bungee jumping, and boxing, solo aerial sports, such as hang gliding and skydiving, and high-altitude activities, such as mountain climbing. People with uncontrolled seizures should also avoid motor sports, horseback riding, gymnastics, ice skating, and skiing.
- Choose milder forms of yoga, such as Iyengar, kundalini, anusara, yin, or restorative, rather than the "hot" power, ashtanga, or Bikram yoga. Avoid Shoulder Stand, Headstand, and any other inversions.

Exercising with a Swiss ball is one of the best forms of strength training for people with epilepsy.

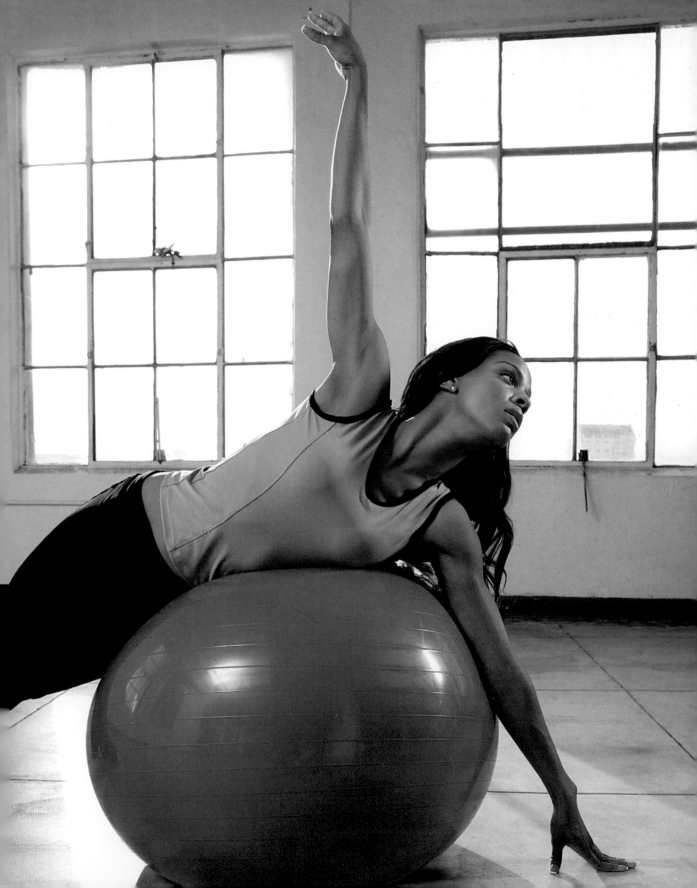

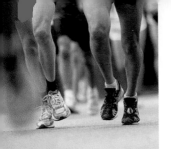

Epilepsy continued

It is rare for a person to have an epileptic seizure while exercising.

Epilepsy drugs and exercise

Anti-epileptic drugs (AEDs) help to manage epilepsy, but they can influence your ability to exercise safely. Some drugs cause fatigue or problems with concentration. Physical exercise can also alter the levels of AEDs in the blood.

People taking AEDs who exercise regularly need to be monitored by their doctor or specialist. AEDs lead to bone loss and a doubling of fracture risk in people with epilepsy. Weight-bearing exercise is a useful preventive for bone loss.

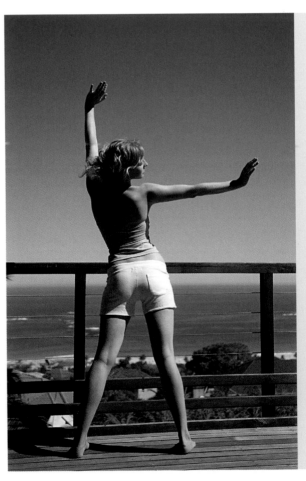

HOW OFTEN?

- Listen to your body. Overexertion or tiredness can trigger seizures in some people, so don't exercise at an intensity that isn't comfortable for you.
- If you are feeling very hot and tired, slow down or stop. Always drink plenty of water before, during, and after exercise.
- A little exercise often, such as 15 minutes of walking or running each day, or a gym session 3 times a week, is better than an extended session once a week.
- Make sure you have at least 2 rest days every week.

A simple qigong exercise to help manage epilepsy

Practice this routine daily for 5 to 15 minutes.

1. *Stand with your feet about shoulder-width apart. In qigong, preparation is traditionally done with your back toward the sun. Position your feet parallel to each other and slightly bend your knees.*

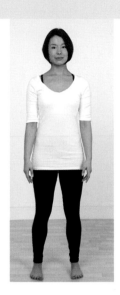

2. *Take a few deep breaths. Instead of allowing your chest to rise, transfer this motion to your stomach. This centers the energy in your body. Repeat a calming affirmation or mantra of your choice to yourself. This helps clear your mind and steady your breath.*

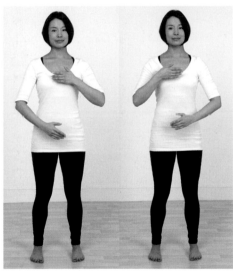

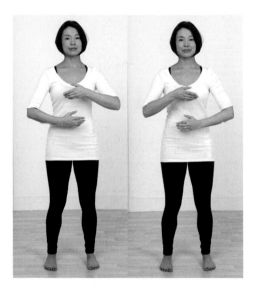

3. *Move one hand up to your chest and lower the other toward your stomach, while focusing mentally on your chosen mantra or affirmation. Exchange hand positions often. By doing this, you are "mixing" the energies from your chest and navel. The movement should be a continuous action with no pauses.*

4. *Visualize the energy flowing within your body, up and down your arms, legs, and chest. You may want to visualize it as colored light. Picture it coming from your hands and moving up and down your body. Continue to say your affirmation or mantra to yourself.*

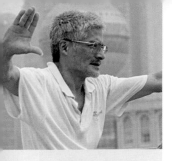

Parkinson's disease

BEST MOVES

balance exercises

qigong

tai chi

stretching

walking

stationary cycling

restorative yoga

aquatic exercise

gardening

Feldenkrais

Parkinson's disease occurs when nerve cells die or become impaired in a region of the brain called substantia nigra. These cells produce dopamine, a chemical that normally facilitates coordination of the body's muscles and movement functions. Once around 80 percent of the dopamine- producing cells are damaged, the physiological symptoms of Parkinson's disease begin to manifest themselves as shaking, slowed movement, stiffness, and difficulty with balance. The disease grows progressively worse and people with Parkinson's in its later stages may fall more easily.

Eventually, the loss of fine motor control makes it difficult to perform everyday tasks, such as getting dressed. Although Parkinson's causes disability, it does not appear to shorten lifespan significantly. Symptoms may fluctuate from hour to hour and day to day, so stop and rest if you feel tired at any point while you are exercising.

Why exercise helps

Exercise can't reverse the symptoms of Parkinson's disease, but it will help maintain functional independence for longer. Researchers at the University of Iowa Hospitals and Clinics studied the role of cardiovascular fitness in Parkinson's disease and found that patients with good cardiac fitness did better on function and mobility tests than those who were not so fit, regardless of their age or the severity of the disease.

Exercise promotes muscle strength, balance, flexibility, and the ability to walk safely and carry out activities of daily living. It can also help with some other Parkinson's symptoms, including constipation, sleep problems, and anxiety or depression. The type of exercise that works best for you depends on your symptoms, fitness level, and overall health. Water exercise, such as aqua aerobics, is easy on the joints, requires less balancing ability, and helps to reduce the fear of falling. Exercises that stretch limbs through the full range of motion are especially encouraged. Some people with Parkinson's have found that the movements used by the Feldenkrais Method, a form of meditative, low-impact exercise (see page 213), have improved their flexibility, balance, and sense of wellbeing.

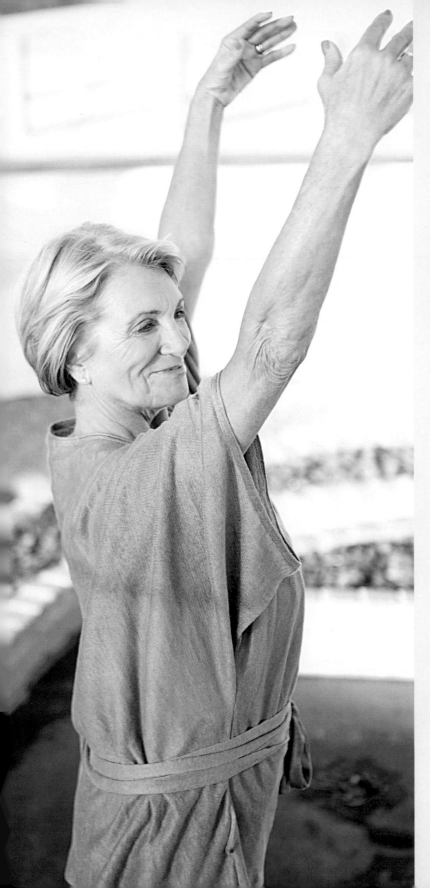

HOW OFTEN?

- Aim for at least 15 minutes of muscle stretches and balance exercises every day. Gradually work up to 40–60 minutes 5 days per week, if possible, alternating a stretch/relaxation session, such as qigong, yoga, or tai chi, with aerobic activity, such as walking, stationary cycling, or aqua aerobics.

- Include a 10-minute warm-up and 10-minute cool-down, such as marching on the spot or swinging your arms. If at any time you feel any discomfort, stop and rest.

- If you suffer from fatigue, try exercising first thing in the morning.

- Qigong is a very gentle practice that is excellent for people with Parkinson's disease.

- Some hospitals and community centers hold exercise classes for people with Parkinson's disease, focusing on stretching. If you go to a class that isn't specifically for people with Parkinson's, always talk to the instructor first about your condition and particular concerns.

Concentration on repetitive physical movements can provide benefits for the brain as well as muscles.

Stretches to stimulate the brain

Repetitive physical movements benefit mental functions, as well as your muscles, by stimulating the central nervous system and enhancing blood flow to the brain. These exercises are also typical of warm-ups at the beginning of qigong, tai chi, and yoga classes. You can also use an elastic exercise band to perform the stretches. Do these exercises between 5 and 10 times for 20 seconds at a time. The stretches can be performed seated if that is easier for you.

HEAD AND SHOULDERS

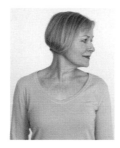 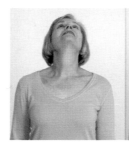 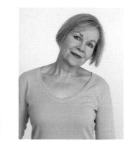

1. *Turn your head slowly from left to right, trying to glance over each shoulder.*

2. *Look to the ceiling, then drop your chin to your chest.*

3. *Drop your left ear to your left shoulder. Straighten up. Drop your right ear to your right shoulder.*

4. *Raise and lower your shoulders. Roll your shoulders forward, then backward.*

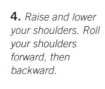 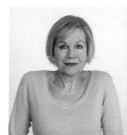 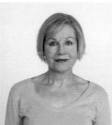 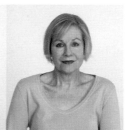

HANDS AND WRISTS

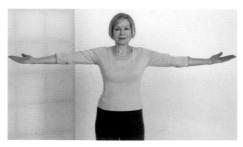 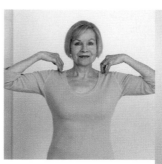 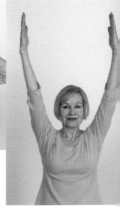

1. *Touch your shoulders, then straighten out your arms to the side, palms facing upward.*

2. *Touch your shoulders again and raise your arms above your head.*

ARMS

1. Stand away from a wall, feet slightly apart and parallel to each other. Press your palms flat against the wall, arms straight, lean in, and stretch.

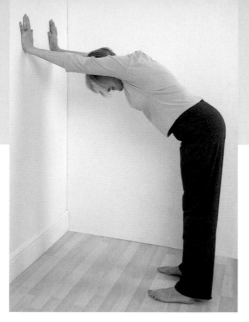

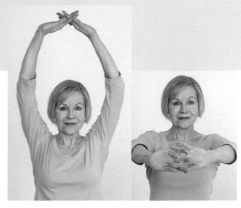

2. Clasp your hands and raise your arms overhead. Then lower slowly.

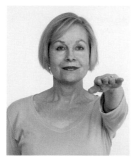

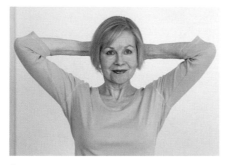

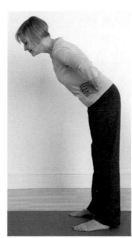

5. Place your hands on your hips and lean forward a little. Straighten up.

3. Stretch out one arm in front of you, then move it to the side. Use a wall or a chair for balance if you need to.

4. Clasp your hands behind your head and open out your elbows.

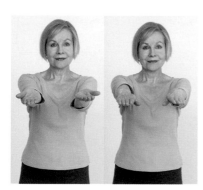

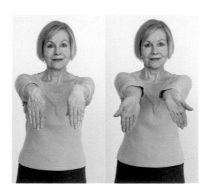

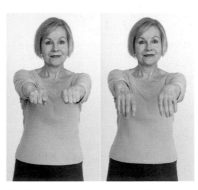

3. Rotate your hands so the palms face up then down.

4. Bend your hands at the wrists, up and down.

5. Clench and unclench your fists.

Muscle stretches continued

LEGS

1. *Lie flat on your back. Bend one knee, and hug it to your chest. Straighten the leg. Repeat with the other leg.*

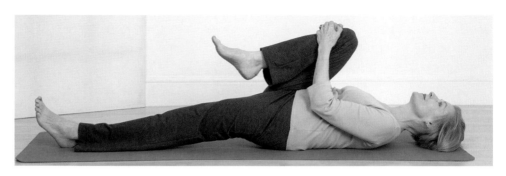

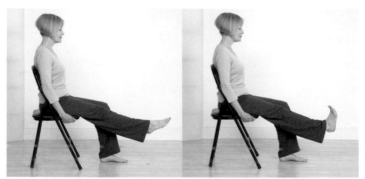

2. *Sit on a chair and extend one leg. Alternately point and flex your foot. Repeat on the other side.*

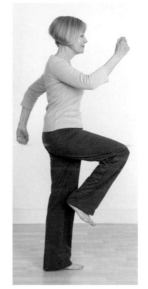

4. *March slowly on the spot, lifting each leg as high as you can.*

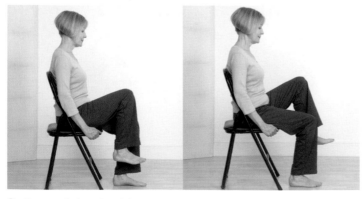

3. *Sit on a chair and straighten one leg at a time. Then slowly raise and lower one leg as if stamping your foot in slow motion. Repeat with the other leg.*

FACE

Exercise your facial muscles, jaw, and voice by singing or reading aloud, exaggerating your lip movements. Make faces in the mirror.

54

Balance exercises

Balance exercises improve stability and can help you avoid falls and broken bones as you age. You can steady yourself while you do these exercises by holding on to a table or wall with one hand. Hold these balances for 5 seconds and repeat the exercises 5–10 times.

FORWARD LEG LIFT

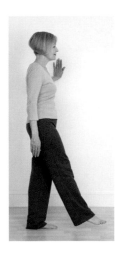

Lift one leg slightly off the floor. Switch to the other leg.

FORWARD TOE TOUCH

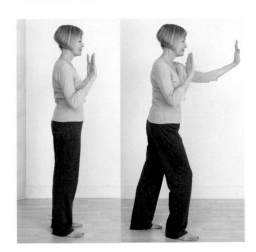

1. Place your feet about shoulder-width apart. Raise your hands to your shoulders with your palms facing forward.

2. Extend your right arm and place your left foot forward, pointing down with your toes and touching the floor. Return to the starting position and do the same with the opposite arm and foot.

STAND ON ONE LEG

1. Place your feet about shoulder-width apart. Extend your arms straight in front of you.

2. Lift your left leg, bend it back, and hold. Change legs. As you improve, practice standing on one leg from time to time throughout the day. The more you practice, the more you'll improve your stability.

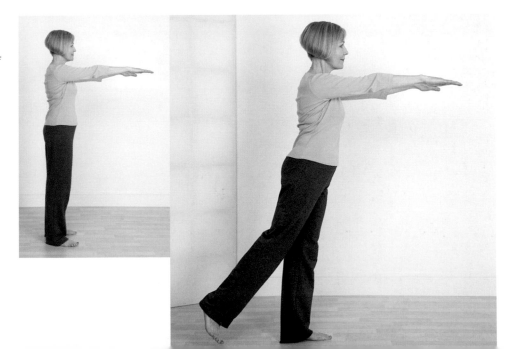

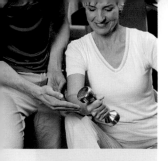

Essential tremor

BEST MOVES

yoga

qigong

tai chi

Pilates

weight training
and resistance
training with
machines

walking

jogging

swimming

cycling

Essential tremor is a disorder caused by abnormalities in areas of the brain that control movement. As a result, the hands and head, and sometimes the arms and legs, tremble involuntarily when purposeful movement, such as writing, pouring a drink, or shaving, is undertaken. It can also affect the tongue and jaw, and the voice can sound shaky. It is not life-threatening, but many people with the condition find the tremors annoying and embarrassing. The shakiness is exacerbated by stress, anxiety, anger, strenuous activity, caffeine, and some prescribed medicines.

Why exercise helps

Physical therapy exercises can sometimes reduce tremor and improve coordination and muscle control. Some people find that exercise aggravates their spasms, but even if this is the case, exercise will still benefit your overall fitness. Your tremor may become more visible post-exercise, but it tends to diminish once you have rested. Exercise is an excellent stress-reliever and a way of lessening anxiety and improving self-image. Weight training and resistance training that strengthen the hands are often helpful for decreasing the magnitude of tremors. Using machines is easier than trying to lift free weights. Cycling on a stationary bike might be less challenging than road cycling.

Yoga, tai chi, and qigong will teach you how to relax and breathe. Yoga will also strengthen your muscles, and qigong and tai chi can improve steadiness. Tai chi and qigong are slow-moving exercises that boost your body's energy, or "qi." Many people have successfully used them for balance disorders. The kind of yoga you do will depend on the severity of your symptoms. You might want to look for a remedial yoga class with a therapeutic program for people with specific health issues.

Self-consciousness

Some people with essential tremor feel uncomfortable at the prospect of exercising in public. If you are struggling with social anxiety, working out at home using instructional DVDs is always an option. Regardless of what you choose to do, stay active if at all possible. If you can find the confidence to go out walking, running, or swimming, or attend a fitness class, you will keep at bay the isolation and despondency that often beset people with essential tremor. Getting out in the open is good for you. Explain to your instructor and

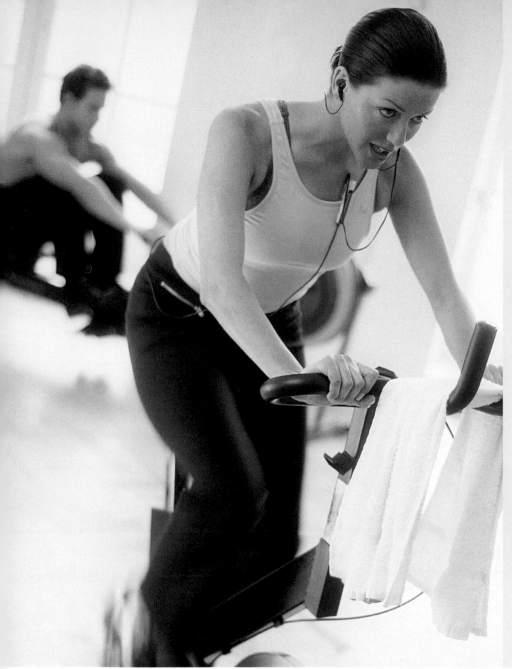

HOW OFTEN?

- The effect of exercise on essential tremor is different for each individual, as is the capacity for different people with this disorder to be able to exercise and for how long.
- Fatigue is a trigger for essential tremor, so be guided by your body. If you are having a bad day, then rest. Otherwise, schedule at least 3 30–60-minute sessions of exercise per week, or walk or jog for at least 15 minutes 5 days per week. If you feel safely able to do more, then go for it!

your fitness companions that you have essential tremor. If you get tired, take a rest. Don't let embarrassment stop you from enjoying physical fitness. You have as much right as anyone to be out in the world, taking care of your health.

Exercise strengthens muscles, which helps to decrease the magnitude of tremors, as well as increasing your confidence.

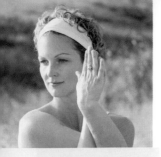

BEST MOVES

yoga

qigong

tai chi

cycling

walking

low-impact aerobics

dancing

stair climbing

aqua aerobics

strength exercises using resistance (elastic) bands

Pilates

pelvic-floor exercises

Feldenkrais

Multiple sclerosis

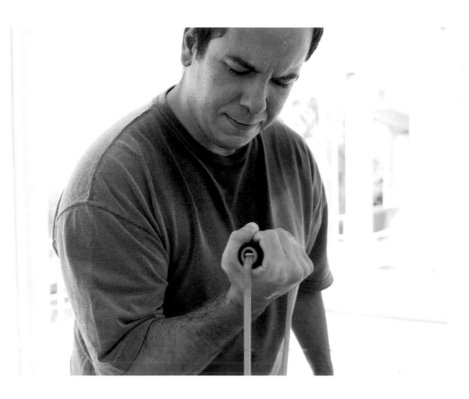

Multiple sclerosis (MS) is a chronic, unpredictable neurological disease that affects the central nervous system. Damaged myelin, the fatty substance that surrounds and protects the nerve fibers in the central nervous system, forms scar tissue (sclerosis) and distorts the nerve impulses, which travel to and from the brain and spinal cord. These distortions produce symptoms that range from mild, such as numbness in the limbs, to severe, such as paralysis or loss of vision. The progress, severity, and specific symptoms of MS can vary considerably from one person to another.

Resistance training of moderate intensity seems to help manage muscle weakness. If you have spasms, pulling an exercise band is easier than using weights.

In the past, people living with multiple sclerosis were advised to avoid exercise altogether, because it was feared that physical activity might aggravate symptoms. In recent years, however, a body of emerging evidence has shown that, far from being detrimental, exercise improves quality of life for people with multiple sclerosis, and can actually help ease symptoms.

Right: *Exercise reduces the weight gain which is a side effect of many MS medications and helps minimize cardiovascular problems.*

Why exercise helps

Multiple sclerosis affects people in different ways, so suitable exercise will vary. If you are severely affected by the disease, work with a physiotherapist to devise exercises that are comfortable for you.

Physical activity can relieve a number of MS symptoms and complications, including fatigue, muscle stiffness, weight gain, brittle bones, mobility issues, depression, anxiety, and difficulties with bladder control. Yoga and cycling have been shown to alleviate fatigue, and weight-bearing exercise helps to build bone density. A study at the University of Tennessee found that twice-weekly 45-minute seated tai chi sessions improved mobility, balance, and stamina. Participants also enjoyed the social nature of the classes.

Exercise also reduces weight gain, which is a common side effect of many MS medications, and helps minimize cardiovascular problems. If your condition alters and you are unable to continue some activities, consult a physiotherapist about new ways to stay active and to find which exercises are most beneficial for you.

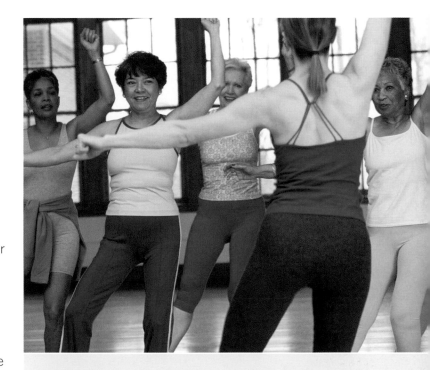

HOW OFTEN?

- At least 20 minutes of aerobic, strengthening, and weight-bearing exercise 2 or 3 times per week, if possible.
- Include one or more yoga or tai chi classes. These usually last 45 to 60 minutes and can be undertaken seated if that is easier for you.
- Warm up with 5 minutes of stretching and range-of-motion exercises—for example, moving the arms, legs, wrists, and ankles in wide-reaching circular patterns.
- Even mild or moderate activity will help. Take it slowly and listen to your body.
- If you experience fatigue or pain during a workout, stop, rest, and seek advice. If your symptoms change, you may need to adjust how much you do.

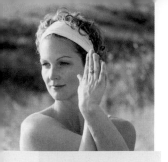

Physical activity can relieve a number of MS symptoms and complications, including fatigue, muscle stiffness, weight gain, brittle bones, mobility issues, depression, anxiety, and difficulties with bladder control.

Multiple sclerosis continued

Exercise for multiple sclerosis

Ask your local MS support group for help in finding classes near you that offer specific exercise sessions for people with mobility difficulties. If there are no such classes in your area, you may find that the instructors at a nearby gym or fitness center would be willing to help you with modifications. Discuss your needs before the start of a class so that the instructor can demonstrate alternatives to movements that might be difficult for you.

Yoga: This encourages flexibility, coordination, and relaxation. It is also easy to modify the postures. Yoga improves posture and keeps your body properly aligned, which reduces strain on muscles and bones. A good teacher will show you alternative postures if you explain your limitations before class. Most styles of yoga, if practiced at a gentle intensity, are helpful for people with MS, except for power, ashtanga, and Bikram yoga. These are "hot" styles, which could exacerbate heat sensitivity.

Tai chi: Many people with MS use tai chi as a way to improve balance and promote relaxation. This ancient Taoist art also helps with blood pressure and heart health. Like yoga, it is easily adapted to the needs of people with MS. Tai chi uses a series of slow, controlled movements to build muscle tone and increase flexibility, and it can be practiced in a wheelchair.

Feldenkrais Method: This gentle technique comprises a series of subtle body movements, which, proponents say, can improve posture, flexibility, balance, coordination, breathing, and performance of different daily tasks that are adversely affected by MS. Some people with MS have found the Feldenkrais Method beneficial, while others have not noticed improvement in their functional performance. There is general agreement, however, that Feldenkrais sessions reduce stress and lower anxiety.

Aquatics: Water aerobics and other aquatic fitness programs are a benign and effective way for people with MS to exercise. Strengthening, stretching, and aerobic exercise can all be done in a pool. Bodies are buoyant in water, which takes weight off the joints and allows for a greater range of movement. Some people who are sensitive to heat may prefer to exercise in cool water. Others may prefer a warm pool.

Weight-bearing exercise: Weakened bones and osteoporosis can be a risk for people with MS who don't get much exercise or have taken long courses of steroids. Gentle activity strengthens the bones and can help prevent these problems from developing. Even if you use a wheelchair, you can undertake some weight-bearing exercise by standing for a few minutes at regular intervals throughout the day, perhaps supported by a frame for balance.

Strengthening exercises: These include lifting and moving small weights, but can also involve using the body's own weight to strengthen muscles and bones. If you have tremor or spasms, pulling against an elastic exercise band might be easier than using weights.

Managing heat sensitivity

Some people with multiple sclerosis are sensitive to heat. If that applies to you, take a cool shower before and after exercising. While you are exercising, sip iced drinks. You also might want to divide exercise sessions into smaller sections, taking regular breaks to stay cool. If you would like to exercise in water, find a pool where the water temperature is below 84°F (29°C).

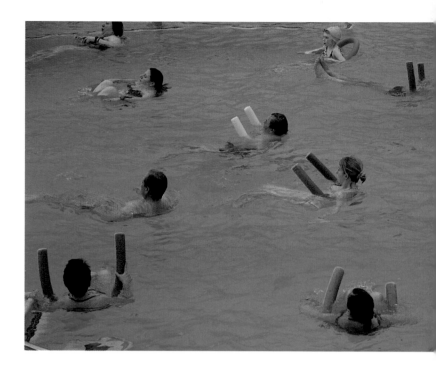

Balance and vision problems

If these make exercise out of doors difficult, you can maybe work indoors on a stationary bike or a rowing machine, with someone in attendance. If you have more strength in your arms than in your legs, a hand-cycle might be an option for aerobic exercise—this is a bike powered by pedals for the hands instead of the feet. You can use a standing frame as an aid to weight-bearing exercise, and weights strapped around the wrists or ankles might help strengthen arms or legs. Trekking poles and walking sticks can help you keep balanced if you do go walking with a companion.

If you are heat-sensitive, keep your core body temperature low by exercising in cool water.

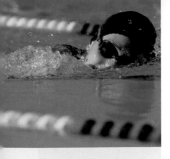

Headache

BEST MOVES

cycling

walking

low-impact aerobics

swimming

Pilates

yoga

tai chi

Tension headaches feel like a tight band is squeezing your head, and the pressure causes a throbbing pain. They can be stress-related or arise from tight muscles in the neck or face, or there may be no obvious cause.

When it comes to headaches, exercise plays a paradoxical role. In most cases, exercise helps to prevent or alleviate a headache, but some people find that sustained exertion causes the abrupt onset of a sharply painful version, known as "exertional" headache. These may follow a bout of strenuous exercise, such as running, rowing, tennis, swimming, weight lifting, or sex. What causes them has not been clearly established, but it's thought that some people react negatively to the dilation of blood vessels that occurs after intense exercise, or to a drop in blood sugar levels. Most exercise-induced headaches are benign and respond to the usual remedies, but if you get one when you're not normally affected, or it is more painful than on previous occasions, see a doctor as soon as possible.

How to avoid exertional headaches

Ease into exercise: Some people find that a change in the weather or in activity can "shock" them into having a headache. No one is quite sure why this is so—it seems to depend on individual brain chemistry—but if you are new to exercise, take it easy at first. Start with a

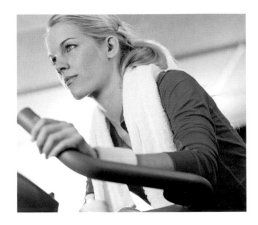

Be sure to build up your exercise routine gradually if you do not exercise regularly so that it is not a shock to your body.

daily walk, rather than a demanding aerobics class, so that your body gets used to it.

Work out in the morning: It's good to wind down during the hours before bed.

Try low-impact exercise: Avoid jarring, high-impact exercise, such as running or kickboxing. These activities are likely to aggravate the pain. Intense exercise will also cause you to sweat, leading to dehydration, which can worsen a headache. Swimming, gentle yoga, and tai chi are most beneficial.

Warm up and cool down: This insures your body does not go through abrupt alterations in heart rate, blood flow, and temperature.

Drink plenty of water: Dehydration can easily trigger a headache.

Don't do inversions: Turning upside down may trigger a headache.

Take an analgesic: Try taking ibuprofen or something similar before you start.

Take a glucose tablet: One of these before you begin will combat low blood sugar. Eat some carbohydrate before exercising and then a meal within an hour of finishing your workout.

Why exercise helps

Even people who have experienced exertional headaches may find that careful attention to exercise may eventually prevent headaches or render them less frequent and less painful. It oxygenates and detoxifies the blood and encourages lymph circulation, which lessens fatigue and promotes wellbeing. Exercise also improves the digestion process and helps your body to absorb more nutrients. Exercise increases production of endorphins, the body's natural painkillers. Endorphin levels are often low in people who suffer from headaches, because of their frequent use of synthetic painkillers. A recent Swedish study showed that indoor or outdoor cycling is particularly effective at reducing the frequency of tension headaches and migraine. Yoga, Pilates and tai chi are also invaluable for correcting the postural problems that cause muscle tension in the back of the neck and provoke tension headaches.

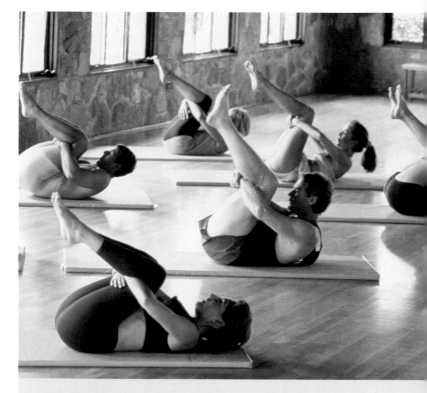

HOW OFTEN?

- If you are susceptible to exercise-induced headache, go slowly. Start by walking or cycling for 10 minutes daily. Gradually increase the duration of the walks or rides, and build up to swimming or cycling at least three times per week for 30–60 minutes.
- If the pounding of running does not aggravate you, try to run three times per week for at least 30 minutes.
- Include slow, deliberate, and meditative exercise, such as Pilates, yoga, or tai chi, at least once a week.

Above: *Exercise reduces muscle tension and anxiety and increases feelings of relaxation.*

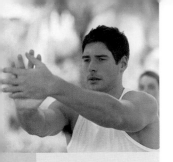

BEST MOVES

cycling

walking

jogging

aerobics classes

swimming

Pilates

yoga

tai chi

Migraine

Migraine is a brain disorder that causes a painful, pounding recurrent headache on one side of the head that can last for hours or days. A quarter to a third of migraine sufferers experience an "aura" before the headache begins, in which a wave of electrical activity travels across the surface of the brain and triggers unusual sensations, such as pins and needles, seeing bright lights, or feeling dissociated from what is going on around them. Women experience migraines more frequently than men do, often as a result of changing estrogen levels.

A wide variety of foods, drugs, environmental cues, and personal events are known to trigger migraines. It is not clear how most triggers set off the physiological events of migraine, nor is it known why particular triggers affect some people but not others. At the onset of a migraine, exercise is ineffective as a relief mechanism, because of the significant pain and nausea of the condition. The migraine sufferer needs to lie down in a quiet, dark room and attempt to sleep. Placing a cold, damp cloth or a cold pack on the forehead may help. Tying a headband tightly around the head may relieve the pain.

By keeping fit, many migraine sufferers find that they can reduce the frequency of chronic attacks. Other preventive measures include eating regularly to maintain blood sugar levels, reducing consumption of caffeine and pain-relievers, refraining from exercise in high temperatures, and getting regular, sound sleep.

Sensitive neurology

Exercise can be an effective preventive measure against migraines for some people, but others find that energetic physical activity actually causes migraines. A study at the Headache Institute at St Luke's-Roosevelt Hospital Center in New York concluded that migraine sufferers have "a heightened neurological system." Their migraines are often triggered by changes to their regular daily routines, such as going to bed late or missing a meal. The Headache Institute suggests that people prone to migraines should establish a schedule not only for eating and sleeping but also for exercising regularly. The tips for avoiding exertional headache on page 62 also apply to migraine. Easing into an exercise program will not "alarm" your neurological system.

Why exercise helps

Individuals with migraine often avoid exercise for fear that it will provoke an attack, but without regular physical activity levels of aerobic endurance decline and general health is undermined. Continuous aerobic activity like cycling can also help prevent

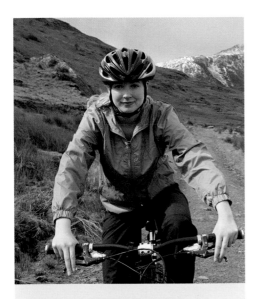

CYCLING DECREASES THE FREQUENCY OF MIGRAINES

A cycling program developed by researchers at the University of Gothenburg in Sweden has improved fitness among migraine sufferers, while proving scientifically that the risk of increased frequency of attacks in connection with this type of exercise is extremely small. Twenty migraine sufferers were asked to undertake regular aerobic exercise by riding on a stationary bike three times a week for three months. The migraine sufferers' maximum oxygen uptake increased significantly. Their migraines did not get worse during the exercise program and during the last month of treatment there was a significant decrease in the number of migraine attacks, the number of days spent with migraine per month, headache intensity, and amount of medication used.

migraines by increasing oxygen distribution, reducing muscular tension and promoting relaxation. Physical activity may also be an effective strategy for some migraine headache sufferers when they experience symptoms that warn them of an impending headache. Even though you may just want to lie down, try moving around and stretching. Try gentle motion exercise such as yoga, tai chi, or slow swimming or if that is too much for you, simply sit with your head relaxed and allow it to dangle with your chin almost touching your upper chest. Turn your head to one side very slowly several times, and then to the opposite side the same number of times. Yoga poses like Shoulder Stand and Fish (see page 68) are also very beneficial because they relax the nervous system. Yogic breathwork, called pranayama, which emphasizes a full diaphragmatic inhalation and exhalation pattern, will also help to establish and maintain a relaxed mind and body.

HOW OFTEN?
- Start by walking, swimming, or cycling for 10 minutes daily. Gradually increase the duration of the sessions and build up to exercise of greater intensity at least 3 times per week for 30–60 minutes. Include slow, deliberate, and meditative exercise in your routine—Pilates, yoga, tai chi—at least once a week.

Stretches to relieve headache

Perform these stretches twice a day in the morning and before bed.

Stretch slowly until the first sensation of stretching is reached, then hold the stretch for 5 seconds.

Relax and repeat 3–10 times.

NECK RANGE OF MOTION

Tip your chin forward to your chest, upward to the ceiling, and then turn your chin to touch each shoulder.

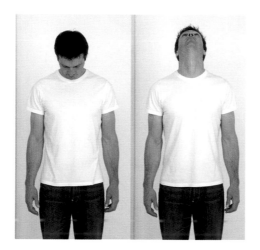 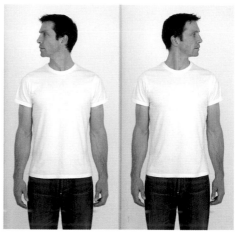

SHOULDER SHRUGS

Shrug shoulders up, then up and forward, and then up and back.

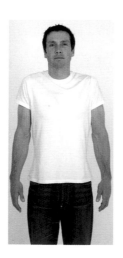 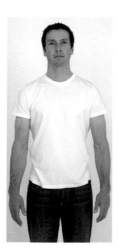 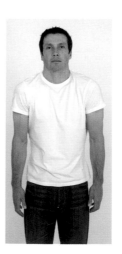 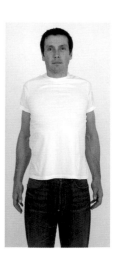

NECK ISOMETRICS

1. *Place your palm on your forehead and press your head against it. Stay still. Don't move your head or hand as you press one against the other.*

2. *Repeat with your hand on each side of the head.*

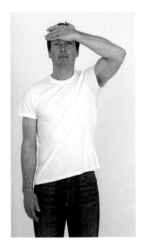

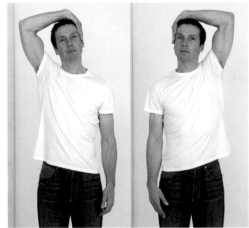

HEAD LIFT

1. *Link the fingers of your hands together and hold them behind your neck at the base of your head.*

2. *Pull your elbows forward and up so you can feel your head lifting up slightly from your neck.*

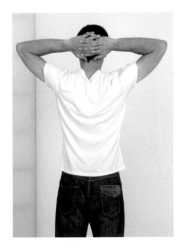

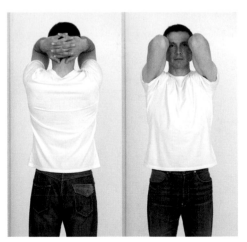

Yoga moves to help migraine

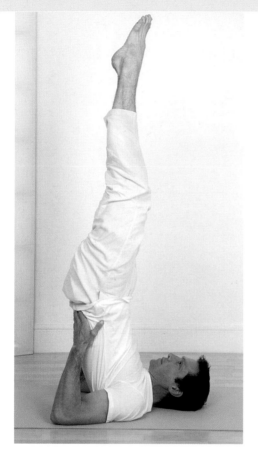

Stress and muscular tension can cause arteries carrying blood to the brain to narrow temporarily. When the arteries dilate again, abruptly increasing blood flow to the head, the sudden shift in blood volume may cause a migraine or severe headache. Yoga poses like Shoulder Stand and Fish help to minimize the muscular tension that causes blood vessels to constrict.

SHOULDER STAND

Lie on your back with bent knees. Exhale, push your feet away from the floor, drawing your thighs into your front torso. As you raise your legs, with toes pointing to the ceiling, spread your palms against your back. Walk your hands up your back to give support while your torso and legs are perpendicular to the floor. Stay in the pose for as long as you feel comfortable.

THE FISH

Lie on your back. Inhale, lift your pelvis slightly off the floor and slide your hands, palms down, below your buttocks. Then rest your buttocks on the backs of your hands. Inhale, lift your upper torso and head away from the floor, then release your head back onto the floor while maintaining an arched back.

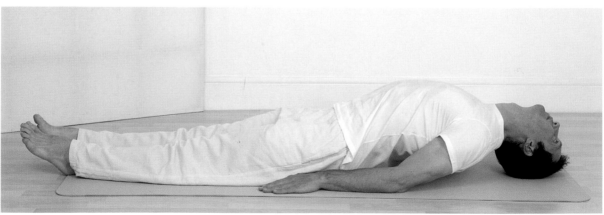

Chapter 4

Your Mind

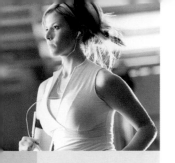

Anxiety and stress

BEST MOVES

walking

running

gym circuit
training

cycling

Nia

dance and
other vigorous
aerobic
exercise

aqua aerobics

yoga

tai chi

Feldenkrais

Stress can arise from any situation or thought that makes you feel frustrated, angry, or anxious. Stress is an inevitable part of life and in small quantities it can be motivating and help you to be more productive. But too much stress can undermine your health and leave you susceptible to infection, heart disease, or depression. Persistent stress often generates anxiety—a habitual feeling of uneasiness or fear that interferes with the way in which you live your life. When we are afraid, our bodies produce adrenaline so that we can either fight the threat or run away from it. If we do neither but remain in an anxious state, adrenaline keeps pumping through our bodies and builds up tension to a point that can feel unbearable. To release this tension, many stressed and anxious people resort to unhealthy behaviors, such as overeating, smoking, or abuse of alcohol or drugs.

Why exercise helps

Exercise helps reduce stress and anxiety before they turn into depression or another serious, incapacitating illness. The feel-good endorphins produced by even one session of aerobic exercise can

Try something different

LINE DANCING

A row of people, all facing the same direction, dance a repeated sequence of steps in unison. There's no physical contact. Line dancing has grown from its country-and-western roots to accompany every kind of popular music style. If it's got a beat, you can line dance to it. It's a great way to have fun in a group without having to have a dance partner.

Line dancing is a great cardio workout, is easy on the joints, improves coordination and mobility, and is suitable for all ages.

BA GUA OR TURNING CIRCLES

Related to tai chi, ba gua is the practice of circle walking as a "soft" martial art. Ba gua martial artists avoid direct attack by moving constantly in circles in varying directions, following the natural ebb and flow of yin and yang energies. Walking the circle tunes into the natural spiraling movements of the planets, stars, and galaxies. The focus on balance, fluidity, and body unity coupled with gentle, low-impact movements makes this an ideal style for promoting healing. And watching the continuous circling, spiraling movements is also a pleasure.

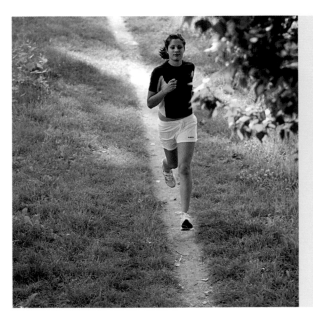

HOW OFTEN?

- Exercise for at least 30 minutes 3–5 times per week. If running, aim for 3–5 miles without stopping. Circuit training should be done 2–4 times per week, with a day off in between sessions to allow your muscles to rest.
- On rest days, walk for 30 minutes. Set small daily goals and focus on consistency rather than perfect workouts.
- Don't turn your exercise into a stress fest or a guilt trip. It's better to take a regular walk for 15–20 minutes than to wait until the weekend for a 3-hour fitness marathon. Lots of scientific data suggests that frequency is most important—and so is enjoyment.

decrease tension, lift and stabilize your mood, and improve sleep. Stress and anxiety can make you feel helpless and at the mercy of external forces, but exercise is empowering. It gives you a sense of accomplishment and that boosts self-esteem. Choose a form of exercise that suits you. Some people like to sweat out stress by running, while others like going to classes with an instructor because it's a relief to have someone else calling the shots for an hour. Yoga and tai chi are excellent ways of winding down.

Vigorous or gentle?

For physical stress symptoms, such as gastrointestinal problems, insomnia, sweating, and palpitations, or aggressive emotions, such as anger and attributing blame, try energetic forms of aerobic exercise. Play tennis, squash, volleyball, or soccer—any vigorous activity that rids your body of stress-causing adrenaline and other hormones.

For stress symptoms that are psychological rather than physical —anxious worrying, feelings of not being able to cope, intrusive thoughts that prevent you from concentrating—it may be better to go for exercises that are calming and make you feel nurtured. Take a walk in the park or the countryside, practice yin or restorative yoga, or try dynamic meditations, such as tai chi, qigong, and kundalini yoga, or trance dancing.

Above left: *Going for a run gives you timeout from your worries, and makes you more resilient emotionally as well as physically.*

Yoga moves to help manage anxiety

MOUNTAIN
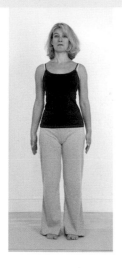
Stand tall with your weight evenly balanced. Firm your abdomen and thigh muscles. Balance the crown of your head directly over the center of your pelvis. Soften your eyes.

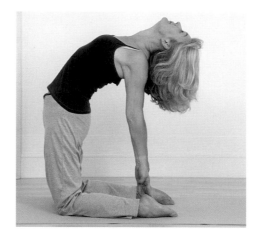

CAMEL
With knees hip-width apart and hands on your waist, extend your spine upward. Lean back slowly and, keeping hips and knees in line, arch your back. Move your shoulder blades down to open your chest. Place your hands on your heels, extend your neck, and look back.

DOWNWARD DOG
Push into your hands and raise your buttocks. Relax the crown of your head toward the floor and release your neck. Keep lengthening the spine and press your heels toward the floor.

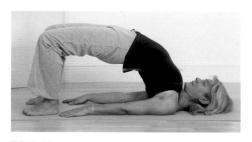

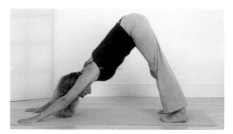

BRIDGE
With feet flat on the floor close to the buttocks and arms extended, palms down, bend the legs. Inhale and as you exhale, push into the palms and heels to lift the pelvis and chest, keeping your chin on your chest.

HERO
From a kneeling position, gradually move your feet wider so your buttocks rest on the floor, but keeping your knees together. Sit back, with your spine straight and your pelvis lifted.

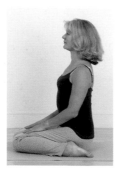

STANDING FORWARD BEND
Stand with feet hip-width apart with your hands on your hips. Inhale, and as you exhale, bend forward, extending your upper body. Let your arms drop to your sides as you go deeper into the stretch. Then, if comfortable, clasp your elbows above your head and let the weight of your arms intensify the stretch.

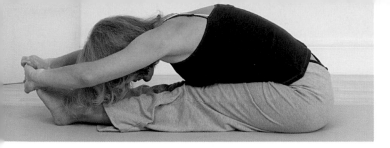

SITTING FORWARD BEND

Keeping your back flat, inhale then exhale as you lean forward and clasp your feet. If you feel comfortable, take your elbows out and bring your head toward your knees. Keep the back of your neck and shoulders relaxed. Press your thighs into the floor.

BUTTERFLY

Sitting comfortably with a straight back, bring the soles of your feet together. Let your thighs drop and relax into the stretch, keeping your neck and shoulders relaxed.

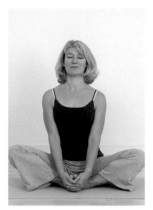

WIDE BEND

Stand straight with legs apart in a V-shape and your feet parallel to each other. With your hands on the outside of your thighs, lift your pelvis and slowly bring your head toward the floor, letting your hands slide down your legs. Place your palms on the floor level with your heels. Breathe into the stretch.

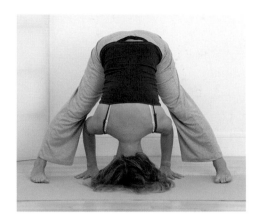

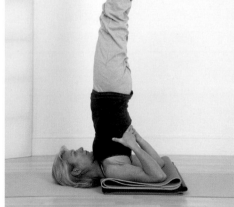

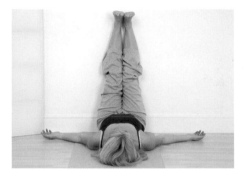

LEGS UP THE WALL

Lie on your side with your buttocks close to the wall. Roll onto your back, and lift up your legs. Take your arms back, palms up, and flex your feet.

SHOULDER STAND

Lie flat on your back, a folded mat under your neck. Inhale and raise your legs toward the ceiling. Place your hands against the center of your back for support, and rest your body weight on your shoulders (not your neck). Keep your spine and legs straight.

BOW

Lie on your stomach, feet hip-width apart and forehead on the floor. Grasp your ankles, taking your heels toward your buttocks. Tuck in your pelvis, inhale then exhale and pull up with your legs, so your back arches and your head and chest lift off the floor. Raise your chin and look up, keeping neck and shoulders relaxed.

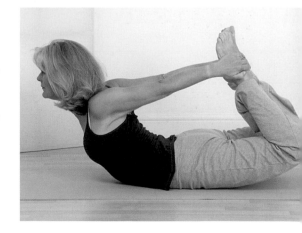

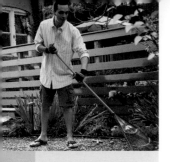

BEST MOVES

walking

running

cycling

Nia

Pilates

dancing

circuit training

yoga

qigong

tai chi

gardening

Depression

A person with depression loses interest in the world and becomes overwhelmed by feelings of helplessness, hopelessness, and low self-worth. Depression manifests itself in disturbed sleep or appetite, low energy, fatigue, poor concentration, and negative thinking that can become suicidal. If you suffer from recurring bouts of depression, your bleak view of the world, and the lethargy that is produced by despair, can make it increasingly difficult to deal with everyday responsibilities.

There is plenty of evidence to show that regular aerobic exercise, especially high-intensity types of exercise, can raise the mood of people with mild to moderate depression, but depressed people often struggle with motivation. It is possible, however, to overcome the inertia of depression by committing to very small amounts of exercise at first—say, for 10 minutes at a time. Choose a form of exercise that really appeals to you and ask a friend to work out with you so that you are encouraged to stick with your routine.

Why exercise helps

Exercise isn't a cure for depression or anxiety, but its psychological and physical benefits can improve your symptoms, and it is an effective way of preventing a relapse after treatment. Even a little exercise helps. It boosts your feel-good endorphins, releases muscle tension, helps you sleep, and reduces levels of the stress hormone cortisol. As these positive physical and mental alterations start to accrue, you may find yourself feeling less sad or hopeless.

If motivation is a challenge, just do something undemanding, such as walking, which requires little skill or concentration and costs nothing. Aim eventually for prolonged exercise that is done in a rhythmic, repetitive manner, such as cycling, running, or long-distance swimming. This kind of exercise is calming and increases production of endorphins.

What an exercise routine will give you

A sense of accomplishment: Even doing just 10 minutes of exercise at a time will make you feel better about yourself, because you have undertaken a positive action and met a goal. If you carry on exercising, it will improve your appearance, too, and that will reinforce a sense of self-worth.

Distraction: Exercise distracts you from the dark subjects and obsessive ways of thinking that stop you from solving problems and making decisions. An expressive activity—dancing, for example—or a fun activity, such as aqua aerobics, can keep you from dwelling on depressed thoughts.

Vigorous exercise distracts you from obsessive ways of thinking and makes you feel better in yourself.

Interaction: Mental health disorders are very isolating and feelings of being alone exacerbate these conditions. Getting involved in exercise classes puts you in an unpressured social situation and gives you a chance to interact with other people, even if it's just saying hello or exchanging a smile.

Green exercise

The benefits of gardening and horticultural therapy have long been recognized as a way of improving mental health, but exercising in a park or the countryside can help, too. According to recent research published by British mental health charity Mind, ecotherapy—being active outdoors in a green environment—decreases feelings of tension and depression.

In a connected study by Britain's University of Essex, 94 percent of participants said green exercise helped with their depression, and 90 percent found that exercise combined with the sensory stimulation of the outdoors, a feeling of liberation, and the spirituality of nature, had a powerfully beneficial effect on their mood.

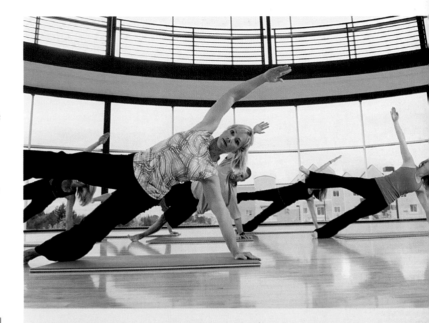

HOW OFTEN?

- Brisk 30-minute walks 5 times per week can help improve moderate to mild forms of depression. Walking for as little as 10–15 minutes at a time can improve mood in the short term. Hour-long exercise sessions 3–5 times per week are another option. To keep motivation high and boredom at bay, alternate different forms of aerobic exercise with an activity that has a strong relaxation emphasis, such as yoga, qigong, or tai chi.
- The important thing is to work out a routine that is realistic and enjoyable for you. If it happens to be half an hour of gardening twice a week, then start with that rather than putting yourself under the pressure of an overly ambitious schedule.
- If you miss a couple of sessions, don't beat yourself up about it. Just try again the next day and give yourself credit for hanging in there.

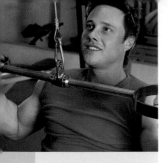

Anger

BEST MOVES

walking

running

cycling

spinning

swimming

weight lifting

boxing

racket sports

capoeira

Latin dance

gym circuit training

vigorous yoga

Anger is a powerful emotion fueled by an adrenaline rush that sends heart rates rocketing. High levels of anger and hostility have been associated with delinquency in children and cardiovascular disease in adults with subsequent risk of heart attack, stroke, and diabetes.

Anger that is not managed is seriously damaging when it is displaced onto family, friends, and colleagues, and manifests itself in aggression and violence. Anger turned inward is also injurious and is often a precursor of depression. The stress of dealing with chronic pain can lead to eruptions of frustration and anger.

The best way to gain control over your anger when you are in a trigger situation is to walk away and take time out. Being committed to a routine of regular exercise makes you less likely to live life as an angry person.

Why exercise helps

Anger often arises from low self-esteem and lack of confidence. Physical activity unleashes endorphins, the feel-good hormones that elevate your mood and make you feel better about yourself. Exercise also acts as a release valve that vents anger and reduces stress responses. Regular high-intensity activities —running, swimming, racket sports, aerobics, dancing, and boxing classes —are effective ways of discharging the pent-up emotions that provoke angry outbursts. Relaxing activities, such as yoga or tai chi, can dispel negative energy and encourage feelings of calm.

HOW OFTEN?

- At least 30 minutes 3–5 times per week.
- If running, aim for 3–5 miles without stopping.
- On rest days, walk for 30 minutes.
- Include yoga or tai chi in your exercise routine to learn relaxing breathing techniques and to keep your body and mind flexible.
- Introduce variety into your routine. Circuit training is a lively, fast-moving way of combining cardio and resistance training, using a repeated sequence of 8–15 exercises performed for a couple of minutes each. Circuit training should be done 2–4 times a week, with a day off in between sessions to allow your muscles to rest.
- As your aerobic fitness improves, extend the amount of time you exercise from 30 to 60 minutes.

YOUR MIND

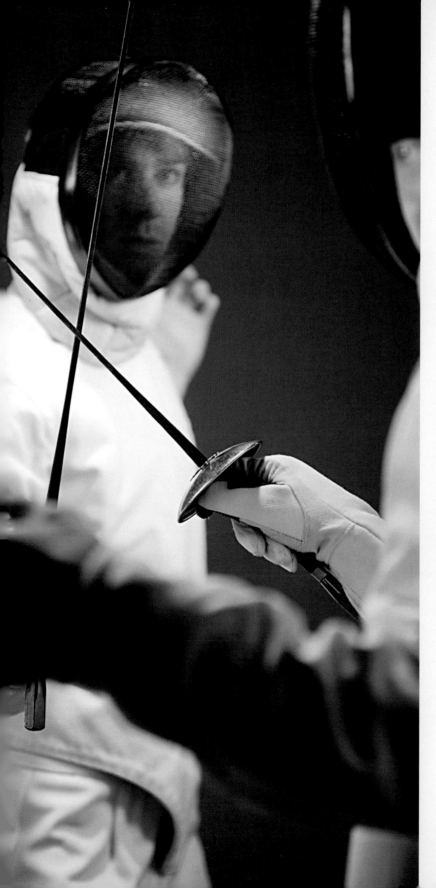

Try something different

FENCING

A fun way to give vent to your competitive nature, this fast-paced, exciting sport increases stamina, strengthens the heart and lungs, and channels aggression in a safe and enjoyable way. The training—try 100 squats followed by 25 full lunges—makes it an incredible workout. Fencing calls for lightning mental and physical reflexes, discipline, adroitness, and endurance. Perfecting fencing's skills is a superb way to cultivate a healthy sense of self-worth and to train the mind to be calm and clear. Also, social interaction with other practitioners of the sport is good for your mental health. New students may be able to fence with each other a few weeks after their first lessons. You can begin fencing at any age.

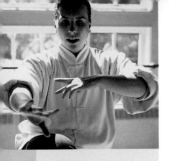

BEST MOVES

walking

running

cycling

spinning

swimming

aerobics classes

circuit training

yoga

qigong

tai chi

Recovery from psychosis

Psychosis is a generic term that encompasses such illnesses as schizophrenia, delusional disorder, bipolar disorder, and depression with psychotic features. These disorders are characterized by disconnection from reality and disorganization of a person's life, emotions, and personality. The exact cause of psychosis is not known. Some people are vulnerable to developing it due to various biological and genetic risk factors, which are triggered by stress.

Exercise has been found to be as effective as traditional therapies, such as psychotherapy and behavioral counseling, for helping recovery, and compared with other interventions can be a low-cost, accessible treatment.

Why exercise helps

Weight gain is a major side effect of the antipsychotic medications used to treat psychosis. The prevalence of obesity among people recovering from psychosis is up to three times that of the general population. These people may also have health issues connected with lifestyle, caused by smoking, poor diet, and lack of exercise. Increasing any physical activity will improve health, quality of life, and feelings of self-esteem, and some studies have suggested a beneficial relationship between structured, supervised aerobic exercise and psychological improvement. In one

study, 78 percent of participants reported that they had used exercise in some way to decrease the prevalence of hallucination, but numbers taking part were small, and the evidence that exercise can reduce symptoms of psychosis is largely too tenuous to be able to make an assertion that this is so.

However, regular exercise has been shown to be a useful therapy for helping people recovering from psychosis to reduce the dosage of their medication and alleviate some side effects. Getting involved in an exercise routine is also valuable because of its social aspect. Going to the gym or a yoga studio helps you feel less marginalized.

Ordering your time and thoughts

Keeping to an exercise routine can help you structure your day and you may find that your thoughts follow suit. Some useful techniques for structuring your time and improving your ability to plan include making lists, using a day-planner meticulously to record appointments, and setting reminders in your phone. Focusing logically on what you need to do takes the pressure off your memory and helps relieve stress. You may like to keep an exercise journal. This can help order your thoughts and show how much progress you are making. The notes can also be used to help your treatment.

HOW OFTEN?

- Lack of motivation is a very common barrier for people coping with mental health problems. If you have been sedentary for a long time, start by walking for 10–20 minutes every day with a companion. You will find it easier to stick with your routine if there is someone to encourage you. Once you build up your fitness you can increase your program to 30-minute aerobic sessions 3 times per week and then progress to 5 times per week.
- If you want to lose weight, you will need to undertake vigorous aerobic exercise 5 times per week for at least 45–60 minutes each session.

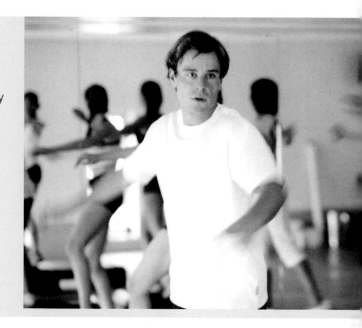

Where to exercise

This is a matter of finding what suits you. Some people recovering from psychosis need to limit stimuli and loud noise, and for them the hectic atmosphere of a gym will probably prove too taxing. If this is the case, the calmer atmosphere of a yoga or tai chi studio may be better. Calorie-burning power yoga or ashtanga yoga are effective for losing weight. Brisk walking in the countryside is another option, or running in the park.

Other people may find that the music and activity of the gym provide a welcome distraction. In this case, try high-intensity classes, such as spinning, boxfit, step, and dance. You may find the loud, upbeat music and the commands of an instructor help to override your internal voices. Going for a run in the early evening may help you sleep.

Try circuit training as well for the variety it offers. Warm up first with a 15-minute walk and gentle stretching. The circuit can include exercises with weights, resistance machines, stationary bicycles, treadmills, rowing machines, exercise balls, and floor exercises. Circuits are arranged so that you don't exercise the same muscle group on any adjacent station. By the time you are tired of one, you are off to another.

However, even if you find you respond to a more intense environment, try to take a qigong, yoga, or tai chi class at least once a week. It will teach you useful stress-reduction techniques.

The structured, high-intensity exercise of an aerobics class may provide a diversion from insistent thoughts and help you to sleep.

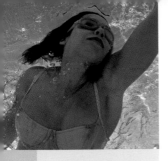

Panic disorder

BEST MOVES

walking

jogging

running

cycling

swimming

rowing

aerobics classes and machines

Pilates

strength training

aqua aerobics

yoga

qigong

tai chi

People who suffer from repeated, unexpected panic attacks, as well as the fear of experiencing them, have a panic disorder. A panic attack is a sudden, intense feeling of terror that triggers the body's fight-or-flight response and causes a rush of adrenaline-induced physical changes, such as a racing heart, sweating, and breathing difficulties.

Sometimes there's an obvious trigger for a panic attack, but mostly the attacks seem to appear from out of the blue. Panic disorder may be accompanied by agoraphobia, a fear of being in places where escape or help would be difficult in the event of a panic attack.

Why exercise helps

If you are someone with "wired-in" anxiety responses, it is possible to bring on a panic attack inadvertently, and some people associate a benign experience, such as exercise, with these attacks. They interpret the elevated heart rate and intensified breathing as symptoms of an imminent attack. Their anxiety triggers fear, which in turn arouses panic responses, further elevates the heart rate, and so establishes a connection between exercise and panic.

For some anxious people, it may take longer than they expect for their heart rate to slow down to normal after exercise. Keep in mind that your heart rate is likely to remain elevated for longer if you are relatively new to exercise and not particularly fit. Regular exercise will develop your fitness and ease general stress levels.

Practicing a meditative discipline, such as qigong, yoga, or tai chi, is an excellent way of learning to manage the

HOW OFTEN?

- If you are not very fit and are also fearful that exercise will replicate the symptoms of a panic attack, begin with a gentle routine. Warm up for at least 10 minutes with stretches, then try 10 minutes of low-impact aerobics, such as walking, cycling, rowing, or swimming, 5 days per week and see how you feel.

- Don't pressurize yourself. Work out for 10 minutes on each of the 5 days for a week. The following week, up the duration of your aerobic exercise to 15 minutes. If all is well, gradually increase it until you are doing 30 minutes of aerobic exercise 5 times a week.
- Take at least one qigong or yoga class per week to learn breathing techniques that will help you to relax.

Slow breathing to help panic disorder

Practice this breathing exercise for 10 minutes after you wake up in the morning and for 10 minutes before you go to sleep at night. If you should feel symptoms of panic, either while you are exercising or in any other circumstances, use these techniques to slow down your breathing and avoid hyperventilating.

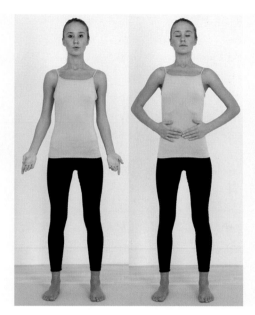

COUNT TO 10
Hold your breath and count to 10. Slowly release your breath.

COUNTS OF 3 AND 10
Breathe in through your nose for a count of 3, then out through your mouth for a count of 3. Continue doing this for one minute. Hold your breath again for the count of 10.

anxiety that lies at the root of panic attacks. If leaving the house is a problem, you can exercise at home with the help of exercise DVDs, or you might consider renting a stationary bicycle.

Keeping calm
Take the time to warm up thoroughly before you begin the more active part of your workout, so that your heart rate is very gradually elevated. Remind yourself that a faster beating heart, and being a little breathless, is entirely normal for someone engaged in exercise.

However, if you are panting heavily during your workout, you are exercising at too high an intensity for your level of fitness. Reduce the intensity of your workouts and focus instead on duration. If running has set off symptoms of a racing heart and hyperventilating, which make you afraid of having a panic attack, limit your aerobic activity to walking on a treadmill until you feel confident enough to begin running again. By undertaking less intense workouts for a time, you will maintain your fitness while "rewiring" your brain so that it doesn't connect exercise with fearfulness.

Exercise to music and use it to distract yourself if you begin dwelling on potential panic symptoms. Cool down with a slow walk around the block or easy pedaling on a bike, followed by stretches.

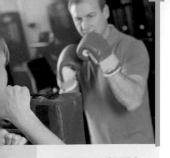

Addictions

BEST MOVES

power walking

running

cycling

capoeira

boxing

dancing

aerobic classes

pump (weight-lifting) classes

vigorous yoga

Dependency on addictive substances is a serious illness, which severely damages the liver, heart, and other vital organs. Alcoholics and drug addicts often die decades before their time, and even in recovery many former alcoholics and drug addicts continue to compromise their health by smoking and overeating. Millions of others struggle to a lesser degree with relapsing into compulsive behavior toward cigarettes, junk food, shopping, gambling, work, or sex, that undermines health, finances, relationships, and self-respect.

Why exercise helps

Exercise facilitates the release of neurotransmitters, such as endorphins and dopamine, which are associated with a sense of reward—the same feel-good factor that addicts look for in their addictive behavior, except that exercise is not deleterious to health. Of course, some people become obsessive

Physical activity spurs changes in the brain that can help prevent addiction to drugs or alcohol.

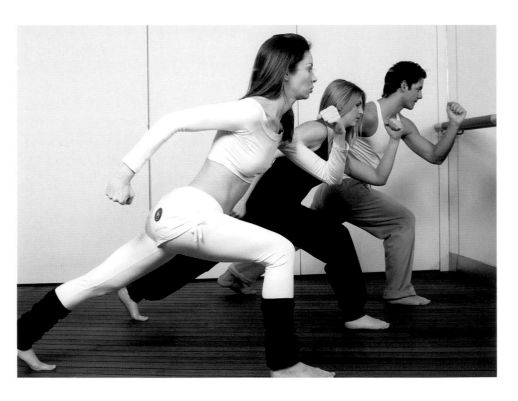

YOUR MIND

about exercise, but there is no evidence to show that recovering addicts are at especial risk of this. In fact, regular exercise has been shown to encourage sobriety, safeguard against relapse, and distract from cravings. Mindful physical exertion can help people with addictions to release tension and work through emotional and mental blocks, as well as improving vitality and self-esteem. Physical exercise also causes alterations in brain activity that can allay nicotine cravings. Researchers at Exeter University in Britain have shown that even five minutes of moderate exercise—taking a stroll around the block, for example—significantly reduces the desire for a cigarette. Another recent study suggests that vigorous exercise may spur regrowth of areas of the brain corrupted by alcohol-induced inflammation. Evidence is also emerging that exercise might play a crucial role in preventing addictions.

Group exercise

Addiction is a lonely and isolating experience. Social interaction is crucial to recovering addicts, who must learn to build relationships without the help of drugs or alcohol. Exercising in a group focused on a healthy activity helps identification with a fresh, more positive community and that is empowering. Boredom, and the fear of empty hours,

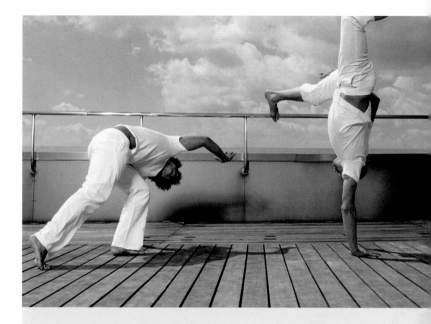

HOW OFTEN?
- **Walk for 10–15 minutes per day, 5 days a week, gradually building up to 30–45 minutes.**
- **Former smokers who get a nicotine craving should go for a walk, run, or bicycle ride that lasts 5–15 minutes.**
- **Once fitness has been established, exercise for at least 5 days per week for 30–60 minutes.**

is an intense stressor for people managing addiction. Joining a running club or a cycling club that schedules regular runs or rides (or committing to a classic six-day-a-week ashtanga yoga practice, for example) is an effective way of keeping boredom at bay.

Above: *Vigorous group exercise like Brazilian dance-martial art capoeira is an empowering way to recover from addiction.*

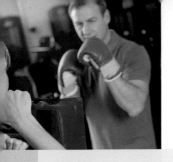

Addictions continued

Mindful physical exertion can help people with addictions to release tension and work through emotional and mental blocks, as well as improving vitality and self-esteem.

Try something different

Anyone recovering from addiction has a void to fill when he or she discontinues the substance or the behavior that has been dominating his or her life. Here are two intense, exhilarating, detoxifying, total body disciplines that are known for their positive, transformative effect on lifestyles and mindset as well as physical prowess.

ASHTANGA YOGA

A set series of poses performed in a flowing, athletic style that combines grace and strength, and develops the ultimate "yoga body." The yoga style most preferred by men. The primary series is designed to detoxify the body, realign the spine, and boost aerobic endurance, flexibility, and mental clarity. Encourages impulse control, peace of mind, and a more positive outlook on life.

What happens in class? Classes begin with warm-up sun salutations and move on to standing and seated poses, inversions, and backbends before relaxation.

How do I start? Join a beginners' class and a teacher will lead you through the primary series. Once you know the order of poses you can go to Mysore-style classes in which you practice at your own pace and level of ability, in the company of other students, supervised by a teacher.

HOW OFTEN?
■ At least three times a week to improve stamina and flexibility. Classes are generally 1 to 1½ hours.

CAPOEIRA

A Brazilian dance-fight discipline performed to music. Combines the grace of dance with the power of martial arts. Develops coordination, aerobic endurance, strength, and a great body. Energetic kicks and twists increase agility, flexibility, and speed. Relieves stress. Imparts a huge sense of fun, sociability, and a sense of belonging to the capoeira community.

What happens in class? Classes follow interval training patterns: cardiovascular sequences mixed with bodyweight resistance exercises and periods of active recovery.

How do I start? Capoeira is open to everyone and is equally for men and women. It has plenty to offer those who are in shape and those who are not. If you are fit enough to get to class, you are fit enough to start training.

HOW OFTEN?
■ Up to three times a week. Like everything, the more you put into it, the more you'll get out of it.

Chapter 5

Breathing

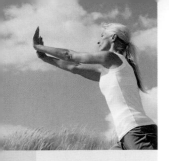

Hay fever

BEST MOVES

swimming

walking

running

cycling

dancing

strength
training

yoga

qigong

tai chi

Hay fever is also known as allergic rhinitis, a condition that affects people who have a seasonal allergy to pollen or mold, and those who are allergic to house dust or furry animals year-round. When you breathe in something you're allergic to, your immune system reacts to the invasion of the pollen, mold, or dust by releasing histamine and other chemicals that inflame the membranes of your nose and respiratory tract. You sneeze and cough, your nose runs, your eyes itch and water. Left untreated, hay fever can cause complications, such as sinus infection, sinus headaches, chronic fatigue, ear infections, and even asthma. You can control hay fever by limiting your exposure to allergens and by treating your symptoms with one of many over-the-counter oral antihistamine medications that are available.

Why exercise helps

Keeping fit is important for your general health, but hay fever can undermine your exercise routine. When you are sneezing and your nose is running, exercise doesn't seem like a very attractive proposition but remind yourself that aerobic exercise will help alleviate your hayfever symptoms. When you exercise, you stimulate the flow of adrenaline, which opens airways and promotes free breathing. By keeping active, you will increase lung capacity and clear nasal congestion, and also help to prevent further complications from hay fever. Many people with hay fever find that swimming is an effective activity because the warm, moist air promotes easier breathing. Some people's hay fever, however, is worsened by exposure to chemicals in swimming pools. There are preventive measures you can take that will enable you to stick with your program even on "bad-pollen" days.

How to minimize hay fever symptoms

When pollen counts are high, you could choose to exercise indoors, either at home or in a gym. But if you prefer to be outside, avoid activity between 5 a.m. and 10 a.m., when pollen counts are highest. Pollen counts have usually fallen by midday, so afternoon and evening are the best times to exercise. Pollen counts also tend to be lower after rain and near lakes, ponds, and rivers.

- Avoid running on windy days. The wind disperses pollen, so run indoors when it's windy.
- Know your personal pollen count. Everyone can tolerate a different level of pollen. Pay attention to the pollen counts and keep track of when you

start to experience symptoms. Then you can choose to run outside when the pollen count is below your tolerance level.

- To prevent symptoms from developing during exercise, take your medication, whether over-the-counter or prescription, about 30 minutes before you head outside to exercise. Warm up slowly.

- If you suffer from dry, itchy eyes during the allergy season, apply eyedrops about an hour before you exercise and wear wraparound sunglasses when you are walking, running, or cycling outside.

- Some people find that wearing a surgical mask or bandana that covers your mouth and nose decreases the amount of pollen that gets into your nose and lungs.

- Most allergy symptoms don't flare up until about an hour after contact with pollen or dust, so while you are exercising outside you may not experience any symptoms. To reduce the risk of symptoms developing afterward, take a shower and change into clean clothes as soon as you get back from exercising.

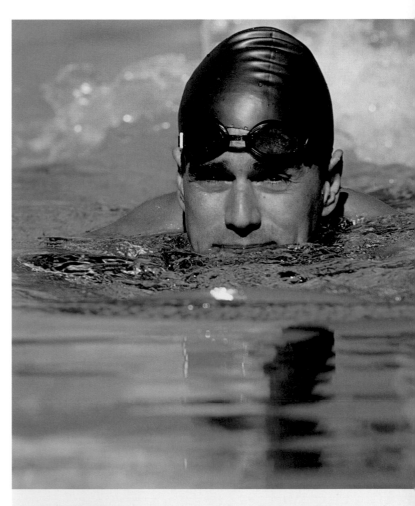

HOW OFTEN?
- **Exercise every day or every other day at least 3–4 times per week for at least 30 minutes at a time unless you are feeling very tired. Fatigue makes your immune system vulnerable.**

Swimming in a heated pool promotes easier breathing for hay fever sufferers.

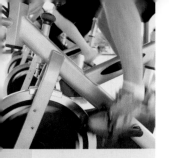

BEST MOVES

walking

swimming

cycling on a stationary bike

climbing stairs

dancing

golf

light weight training for the upper body

gentle yoga

qigong

tai chi

Chronic obstructive
pulmonary disease

Chronic obstructive pulmonary disease (COPD) is a general term used to describe a condition that involves chronic bronchitis or emphysema, or both. People with COPD have airways that are permanently damaged, usually because of smoking. Obstructed airflow to the lungs causes coughing, breathlessness, and chest infections. Inhalers are commonly used to ease

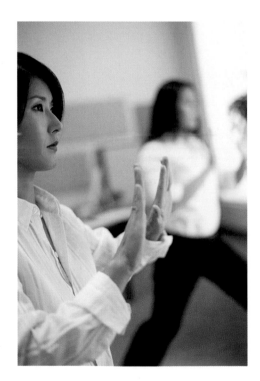

Regular tai chi can help chronic obstructive pulmonary disease. Practicing outdoors in the fresh air will also benefit the body.

symptoms, but there is no cure for COPD. As the disease progresses, mobility and general quality of life may become poor due to increasing breathing difficulties. There is also a risk of heart failure. The most important treatment is to stop smoking. Any damage already done to the airways cannot be reversed, but stopping smoking prevents the disease from getting much worse. In addition to medication, people with COPD can help manage the disease by having an annual shot to immunize against influenza. Losing weight and undertaking regular exercise are also helpful.

Why exercise helps
Many people with COPD avoid physical activity because they associate it with breathlessness, muscle fatigue, or tiredness, but exercise and staying active help significantly in the rehabilitation of chronic lung disease. Exercise can't reverse COPD, but it can improve physical capacity. Regular exercise tends to improve breathing, ease symptoms, strengthen the heart and cardiovascular system, and build energy levels, which makes for a better quality of life. People with COPD who exercise regularly improve their endurance levels and can do more with their limited lung capacity. The more you exercise, the easier routine activities

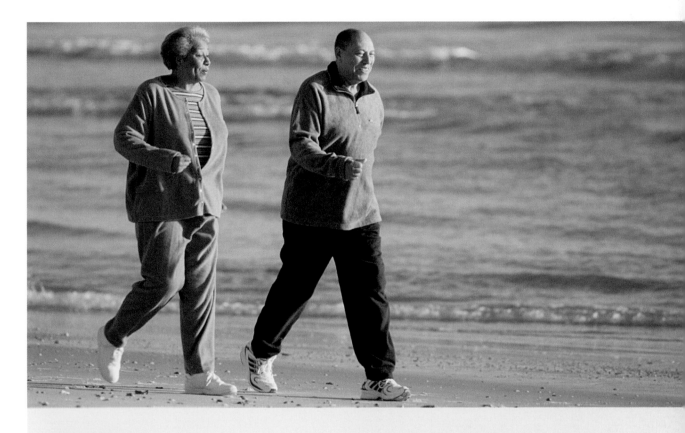

HOW OFTEN?

- Start by walking 3 times daily for 5–15 minutes at a time. Walk at a pace that causes moderate breathlessness. Take regular rests if you are very breathless or tired, recover by doing pursed-lip breathing (see page 91), and then begin walking again. Gradually build up to walking for 30 minutes on at least 5 days each week.
- Once you have built your fitness base by walking, aim to exercise for at least 30–45 minutes on 5 days a week, or every other day. Whatever exercise you do, it should make you a little out of breath.

- Your sessions should include aerobic exercise as well as strength training. Aerobic exercise improves cardiovascular fitness and allows your body to use oxygen more efficiently. Swimming, walking, climbing stairs, and dancing are all great aerobic exercises. Begin with a 5-minute warm-up, including stretching exercises, before any aerobic activity and include a 5–10-minute cool-down after the activity.

Above: *Walking is a good way to build up your fitness, but be careful not to push yourself too hard.*

89

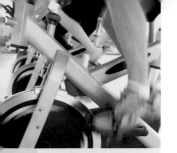

Chronic obstructive
pulmonary disease continued

People with COPD who exercise regularly improve their endurance levels and can do more with their limited lung capacity.

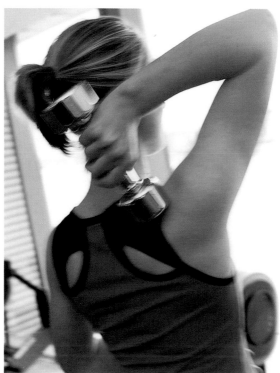

Simple strengthening exercises for the upper body condition the muscles around the shoulders and upper arms that help with breathing.

become. Exercise will help you to keep your weight under control, too. Excess fat, especially around the stomach, presses on the diaphragm, making it harder to breathe.

Regular exercise can help people with COPD reduce anxiety and depression. One reason for the decrease in anxiety may be that exercise

Exercises to avoid when you have COPD
- Avoid push-ups, sit-ups, and isometric exercises—these involve pushing or pulling against an immovable object, such as a wall or a bar.
- Heavy lifting or pushing.
- Tasks such as shoveling, mowing, or raking.
- Outdoor exercises when the weather is very cold, hot, or humid.
- Walking up steep hills.

desensitizes you to the shortness of breath that you live with on a daily basis. You may come to see that you can become short of breath during exercise without any negative effects.

A regular walking program is the most effective way to begin building fitness. When the weather is inclement you can continue to walk on a treadmill at a gym, or perhaps rent a treadmill or stationary bike so that you can exercise at home. Swimming is also very helpful for people with COPD. Simple strengthening exercises for the upper body are useful for conditioning the muscles around the shoulders and upper arms that help with breathing. Work with light weights only at a gym.

Qigong and tai chi, two practices that use deep breathing and meditation techniques, are beneficial for people with COPD. The breathing techniques and postures of yoga are also particularly rewarding for respiratory health. Poses that engage the chest, shoulders, neck, torso, pelvis, and spine will improve the strength and efficiency of the breathing muscles. Forward bends help you exhale more completely and strengthen the expiratory muscles. It is helpful to coordinate breathing with movement. As an example, exhale while bending forward and inhale when you come back up, taking a longer time on the bending forward exhale. Simple backbends, such

Pursed-lip breathing
This technique can help improve lung function before starting exercise. Pursed-lip breathing helps change pressure in the airways and prevents small airways from collapsing. When you experience shortness of breath during an activity, this is an indication that your body needs more oxygen. If you slow your rate of breathing and concentrate on exhaling through pursed lips, you will restore oxygen to your system more rapidly than would otherwise be the case.

- Inhale through the nose, moving the abdominal muscles outward so that the diaphragm lowers and the lungs fill with air. Keep your mouth closed as you inhale, which warms the air you are breathing in.
- Exhale through the mouth with the lips pursed, making a hissing sound.
- Try to inhale for two seconds and exhale for four seconds. You might find slightly shorter or longer periods are more natural for you. If so, just try to breathe out for twice as long as you breathe in, so that pressure is experienced in the windpipe and chest, and trapped air is forced out.

as the beginning of Sun Salutations and Cobra pose, are good for the chest muscles. Side bends, such as Triangle pose, and spinal twists are helpful for strength and flexibility of the rib cage and for improving the capacity for side-rib diaphragm breathing. Yoga also promotes relaxation and emotional calm.

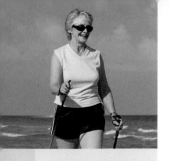

BEST MOVES

swimming

walking

cycling

Pilates

yoga

qigong

tai chi

volleyball

baseball/softball

running on a treadmill

Asthma

Asthma is a chronic disease in which the small airways within the lungs narrow as a result of inflammation and muscle spasm. The symptoms, which can vary from mild to life-threatening, are shortness of breath, tightness in the chest, wheezing, and coughing. The cause of asthma is not known, and currently there is no cure. It is controlled by avoiding triggers and by taking medication.

Some triggers are allergies and environmental sensitivities specific to an individual person, and others are more general, such as exercise. In approximately 80–90 percent of people known to have asthma, attacks can be exercise induced. Ten percent of the general population has an unrecognized history of chronic asthma. These people experience symptoms only during exercise.

Exercise-induced asthma (EIA)

Whether exertion brings on an asthma attack depends on the type of exercise, its duration and intensity, and how sensitive your bronchial tubes are. It also depends on the temperature. Cold, dry air frequently sets off an asthma attack. If you run in cold air, for example, the

The calm and curative Downward Facing Dog is a yoga pose that is beneficial for people with asthma.

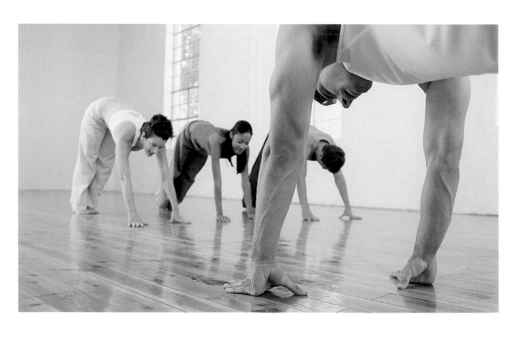

intensified breathing caused by the exertion cools and dries the lining of the bronchial tubes. This cooling produces chemicals that irritate and constrict sensitive airways. A swim in a heated pool, however, is unlikely to trigger asthma, because the humid air helps to keep the airways open. Chlorine and swimming in cold water can trigger some people's asthma, though. Gentle exercise, generally, is better for asthma sufferers than strenuous exercise, as are sprint rather than endurance events.

Controlling EIA

A proper, careful warm-up before exercising, in conjunction with taking the relevant medication, can help reduce or even prevent EIA. An attack will usually respond to rest and the inhalation of reliever medications. Very occasionally, an attack of EIA is severe, in which case supplemental oxygen and larger doses of reliever medications may be called for. An Indiana University study found that the ingestion of caffeine (about the amount in a regular cup of coffee) within an hour of exercise can reduce symptoms.

Why exercise?

One of the goals of asthma treatment is to help you keep up a normal lifestyle, which includes exercise and

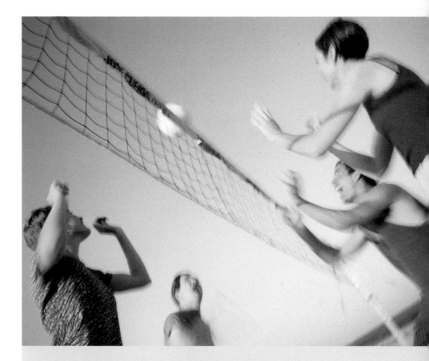

HOW OFTEN?

- Increase your fitness levels gradually. Aim to exercise 3–5 times per week for at least 30 minutes per session, but note that the 30 minutes is best made up of short bursts of exercise if you have previously experienced exercise-induced asthma. Short bursts of exercise of less than two minutes are less likely to cause an asthma attack than prolonged exercise.
- Go for activities that involve intermittent periods of exertion such as volleyball or baseball/softball. If your asthma is not exacerbated by exercise, aim for 20–30-minute sessions of aerobic exercise 3–5 times weekly.

Above: *Stop-start activities like volleyball are less likely than endurance workouts to trigger an asthma attack.*

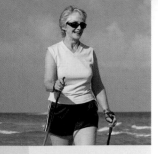

Asthma continued

other physical activities. Maintaining an active lifestyle is important for both physical and mental health. Although exercise can trigger asthma attacks in some people, studies have shown that exercise improves cardiopulmonary fitness in people with asthma. It increases the ability to take up oxygen and improves ventilation. No evidence has been found to suggest that regular exercise worsens asthmatic symptoms.

What this means is that people with asthma don't have to avoid regular physical activity. If asthma symptoms prevent you from participating fully in activities, talk to your doctor. A small change in your treatment plan may be all that is needed to provide asthma relief during exercise. If your asthma is under control, you should be able to take part in any sport or exercise that you enjoy.

PRECAUTIONS

If you have experienced episodes of exercise-induced asthma, ask your asthma nurse to measure your lung function with a peak-flow meter, or spirometer, in order to establish whether you remain at risk of another attack. If lung function remains below 80 percent of personal best after the use of pre-exercise medication, vigorous exercise should be postponed.

- Some exercise is too risky for people with asthma. Do not scuba dive, for instance. The compressed air breathed during scuba diving is cold and dry with the potential to provoke asthma. Climbing, hiking, and skiing at high altitudes, or in cold weather, can also cause problems.

- Make sure the people you are exercising with know you have asthma.
- If the weather is cold, exercise indoors or wear a mask or scarf over your nose and mouth.
- Warm up and cool down thoroughly to help prevent the abrupt changes that can trigger symptoms.
- About 10–15 minutes before you begin to warm up for exercise use your reliever inhaler (bronchodilator) which will relax the muscles around the bronchial tubes.
- Keep a reliever inhaler with you in case asthma symptoms develop while you are exercising. If they do, stop and inhale your quick-relief medication. Once your symptoms have completely gone, restart the exercise.

Warm-ups for people with asthma

Your warm-up should last for 10–15 minutes. First, breathe in for the count of 3 and out for a count of 3 for a minute.

1. *March on the spot, swinging your arms vigorously.*

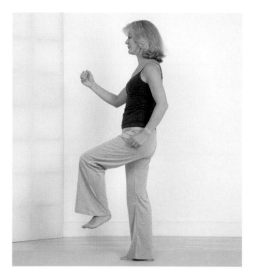

2. *Up the tempo to a jog.*

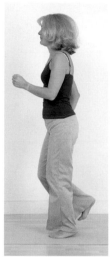

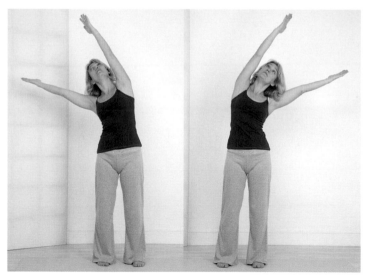

3. *Stand with feet shoulder-width apart and reach both arms overhead. Stretch to the left and to the right.*

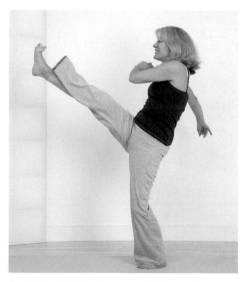

4. *Perform kickboxing moves, kicking to the front and to the rear and then to each side, for several minutes.*

Yoga poses to help relieve asthma

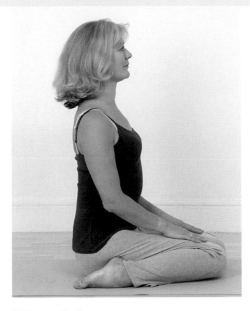

Sitting on Heels

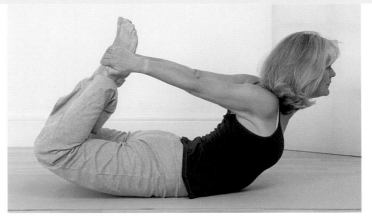

The Bow

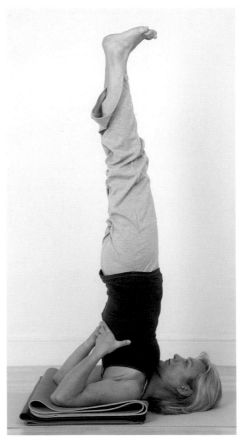

Shoulder Stand

If you suffer from asthma, choose yoga poses that expand the lungs and open up the chest cavity, such as Sitting on Heels (see page 72) and the Bow (see page 73), and inverted positions, such as Shoulder Stand (see page 73) and Plow (see page 150).

Chapter 6

Bones, Joints, and Muscles

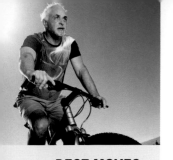

BEST MOVES

aqua exercise

stretching

tai chi

strength training

walking

cycling

stair climbing

elliptical trainer

gentle yoga

qigong

Arthritis

Arthritis refers to a group of more than 100 rheumatic diseases and other conditions that can cause pain, stiffness, and swelling in the joints, and decreased function. The incidence of arthritis increases with age, but nearly three out of every five sufferers are under the age of 65. The two most common types of arthritis are osteoarthritis and rheumatoid arthritis.

Osteoarthritis is a degenerative disease that results from wear and tear of the joints, usually the knees, hips, hands, and spine. It is a major cause of disability. There are currently no drugs available that slow down its progression, and the only treatment is symptom relief, and ultimately joint replacement.

Rheumatoid arthritis is an autoimmune disease that occurs when the body's immune system attacks the cell lining inside the joint. It causes swelling that can lead eventually to deformity. Sometimes symptoms make even the simplest activities, such as buttoning a shirt or taking a walk, difficult to manage. There is no cure for rheumatoid arthritis.

Why exercise helps

Mild, regular exercise can help strengthen the muscles around the joints, improve flexibility, reduce pain, ease sore, stiff muscles, and give you more energy. Activity also keeps cartilage (the tissue that covers the ends of bones in a joint) in good condition, by stimulating the production of fluid around the joint. Even exercising as little as one hour and 15 minutes a week will make a difference. Consult a physiotherapist or a fitness instructor experienced at working with people with arthritis to establish what intensity of exercise is appropriate for you.

Exercising in buoyant, heated water is an ideal way for people with arthritis to maintain fitness, although the temperature of the water needs to be high—89.6°F (32°C)—which is much warmer than most public heated pools. Gentle yoga and tai chi are also helpful for improving pain and disability among arthritis sufferers. Check with relevant organizations for exercise classes in your area that are specifically geared to people with the disease. You can also buy DVDs that demonstrate exercises suitable for people with arthritis.

Stretching

Have a warm bath or shower before and after stretching. Gently straightening and bending the joints in knees, hands, and fingers can help condition them and prevent permanent loss of mobility. Stretching also helps you relax and release tension. Range-of-motion exercises, such as raising your arms over your head or rolling your shoulders

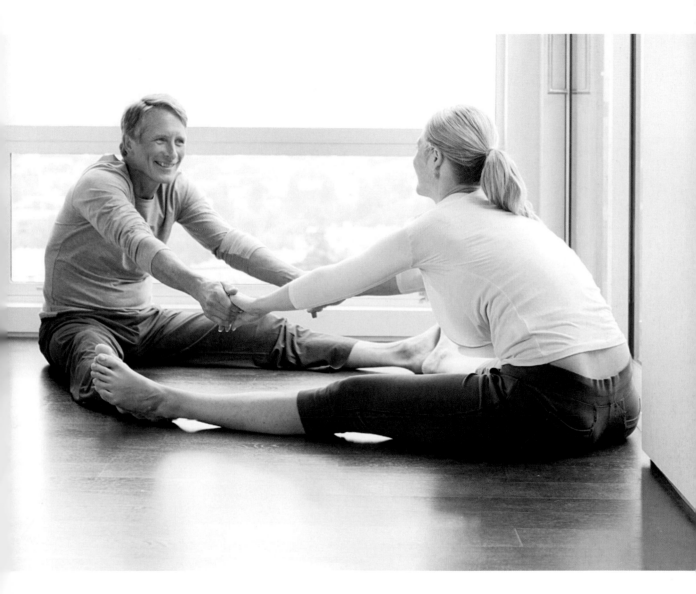

forward and backward, are important as a warm-up for strength and endurance exercises. You can also do your stretching exercises supported by the warm water in a swimming pool.

Beginner yoga and tai chi classes provide simple, gentle movements that gradually build strength, balance, and flexibility—all elements that may be especially beneficial for people with

Regular stretching helps prevent permanent loss of mobility.

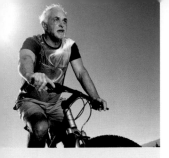

Consult a physiotherapist or a fitness instructor experienced at working with people with arthritis to establish what intensity of exercise is appropriate for you.

Arthritis continued

arthritis. Don't forget to tell your instructor about your condition, though, and be cautious with movements you haven't tried before.

Strength training

Strong muscles help stabilize weak joints and one way to strengthen muscles is through isometric exercise, also known as static strength training, which uses resistance. With this technique, you can tense muscles without any visible movement, and without stressing the joint—by pushing against a wall or door frame, for example. Holding small dumbbells or stretch bands in a fixed position has a similar effect.

You can also use the resistance of your own body to help strengthen muscles. For an isometric chest press, hold your arms at chest height, press the palms of your hands together, and hold for five seconds. Rest for five seconds. Repeat the palm press five times.

Isotonic exercises strengthen the muscles by moving the joint. Straightening your knee while sitting in a chair, for example, helps strengthen your thigh muscle.

Endurance activity

Aerobic, or endurance, activity increases the efficiency of your heart, lungs, and muscles, and develops stamina. Low-impact activities, such as walking,

cycling, stair climbing, working out on an elliptical trainer, and water exercises, are easy on the joints and help build strong bones.

Tai chi for arthritis

Over the last several years, a number of tai chi programs have been designed specifically for people with arthritis. They use just 12 movements or positions to ease pressure on the joints and encourage mobility. Classes begin with warm-up exercises. The instructor then demonstrates one or two movements, which you practice and memorize, and the lesson ends with cool-down exercises.

Aqua exercise

The soothing temperature and buoyancy of warm water make it an ideal medium for people with arthritis to use to maintain fitness. Aqua exercise relieves pain and stiffness, while at the same time providing resistance training. The cushioning effect of water makes exercising gentler on the body while still giving you a thorough workout.

Opposite: *Aquatic exercise uses the natural resistance of water to build muscle strength. Walk around the pool, swinging your arms as you go and stopping every so often to hug each knee in turn to your chest.*

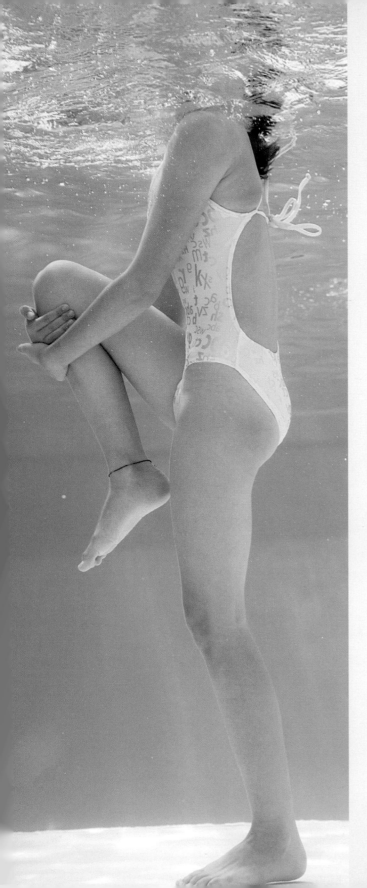

HOW OFTEN?

- **STRETCHING** Warm up with 10 minutes of walking before doing up to 15 minutes of stretching and flexibility exercises daily. Hold stretches for 30 seconds at a time. Squeezing a soft ball, about the size of a tennis ball, helps to keep wrists and hands mobile. Once you can do 15 continuous minutes, start to add strengthening and aerobic exercises to your routine.

- **STRENGTHENING** Do strengthening exercises for up to 15 minutes every second day after warming up with flexibility exercises. Include resistance exercises 2 or 3 times a week, using elastic bands, free weights, or machines.

- **AEROBIC ACTIVITY** Try to perform about 15–20 minutes of activity that increases the heart rate at least 3 times per week, gradually building up to 30 minutes daily. Split that time into 10-minute blocks if that's easier. Use stretching exercises to warm up first for 5–10 minutes and cool down afterward for the same amount of time. Exercise in a heated pool for up to 45 minutes 2 or 3 times per week.

- **TAI CHI** If you are practicing tai chi to manage arthritis, you will need to attend a class once or twice a week and practice a few movements for about 10–15 minutes each day. If you learn at home, you can set your own pace. Gradually build up your practice sessions and aim for about 10–20 minutes of tai chi on most days.

Exercises to help arthritis

SHOULDERS

Forward arm reach:
Raise one or both arms forward (keeping them submerged at this stage) and then upward as high as possible. If one arm is very weak, you can help it with the other arm.

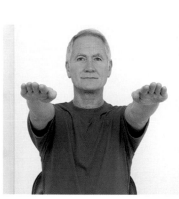 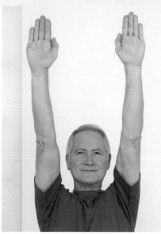

Side arm reach: *Slowly raise both arms out to the side, keeping the palms down and the arms submerged in the water. Lower arms.*

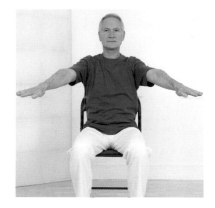 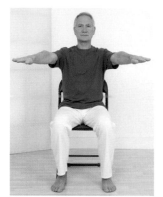

Arm circles: *Raise both arms forward until they are a few inches below the surface of the water. Keep elbows straight. Make small circles with the arms. Gradually increase circle size while keeping the arms beneath water level. Then decrease the circle size. Make inward, then outward, circles.*

ELBOWS

Elbow bend: *Bend the elbows and touch thumbs to the shoulders. Relax elbows and straighten your arms at your sides.*

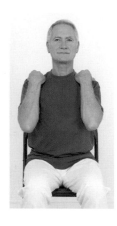

Elbow bend, arms turned: *Hold the arms straight in front of you, hands up, palms facing forward. Bend the elbows until fingertips touch shoulders. Relax and straighten your elbows.*

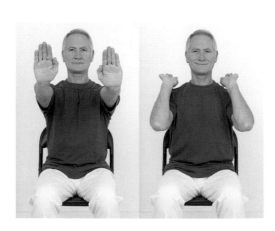

The following exercises can be done at home, or while sitting in a spa or sitting or standing in a pool—make sure that you submerge the part of the body you are exercising.

WRISTS AND FINGERS

Wrist turn: *Hold the arms straight in front of you, palms toward the ceiling. Then turn palms down to face the floor or the bottom of the spa or pool.*

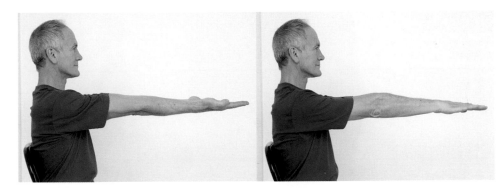

Wrist bend: *Hold the arms straight in front of you and bend wrists backward and then forward.*

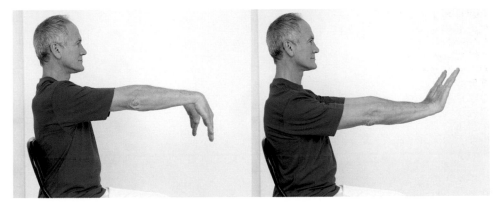

HANDS AND FINGERS

Finger hold: *Touch the tip of the thumb to the tips of the fingers on the same hand, one at a time, to form a round letter "O." Repeat with the other hand. If you like, you can do this simultaneously with both hands.*

Finger curl: *Curl the fingers into the palm to make a loose fist, then straighten them out.*

Thumb circles: *Move the thumb in a large circle, forward and backward.*

ANKLES AND TOES

Ankle bend: *Sit with back supported and slowly straighten one knee. Bend the ankle and point the toes. Then flex the foot so toes point toward the ceiling. Repeat with the other leg.*

Toe curl: *Curl right toes down and then straighten them. Repeat with left foot.*

Ankle circles: *Sit with back supported and slowly straighten one knee. Make large inward, then outward, circles with the foot, moving from the ankle. Repeat with the other foot.*

Exercises to help arthritis

HIPS AND KNEES

Knee bend: *Sit with back supported and slowly raise one foot, straightening the knee. Hold for 3 seconds.*

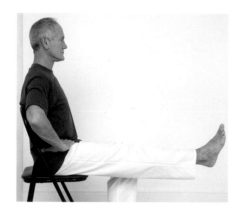

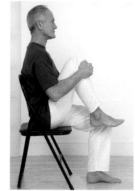

Knee to chest: *Sit straight. Lift one knee and hug toward chest, hands under the thighs or over the knee to assist with the stretch.*

Spread eagle hip: *Sitting on the edge of the seat, straighten one knee. While holding it straight, slowly move it out to the side, hold for 3 seconds, then bring it back to the center. Repeat with the other leg.*

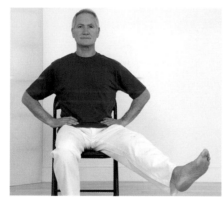

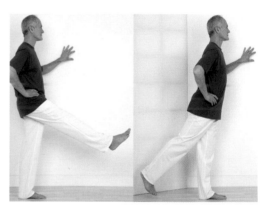

Knee lift: *Stand with left side to a wall, or the side of a pool, holding wall with left hand for balance. Bend right knee, bringing thigh parallel to the floor, or water surface. Straighten the knee; then bend it again. Lower the leg, keeping knee bent. Repeat with the other leg.*

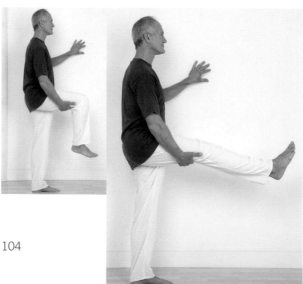

Leg swing: *Stand with left side to a wall, or the side of a pool, holding wall with left hand for balance. Keeping knees straight, lift right leg slowly forward to a comfortable height. Hold for a count of 5 seconds, if possible, then slowly swing the leg backward, using the hip only. Waist and neck should remain still. Keep the upper body straight. Repeat with the other leg.*

Calf stretch: *Stand with left side to a wall, or the side of a pool, holding wall with left hand for balance. Stand straight with legs slightly apart and left leg forward. Keeping body straight, lean forward, slowly letting left knee bend. Keep right knee straight and heel flat. Hold for 5 seconds. Return to starting position. Repeat with right leg forward.*

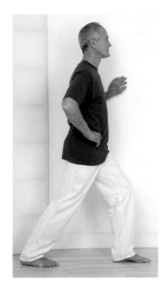
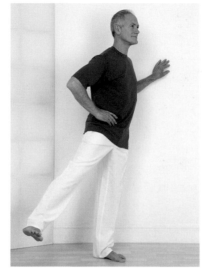

Side leg lift: *Stand with left side to a wall, or the side of a pool, holding wall with left hand for balance, knees relaxed. Swing right leg out toward center of pool and back to midline. Repeat with other leg.*

TRUNK

Side bend: *Place hands on hips and, without moving your feet, bend slowly toward the right; then return to starting position and bend to the left. Do not twist or turn the trunk.*

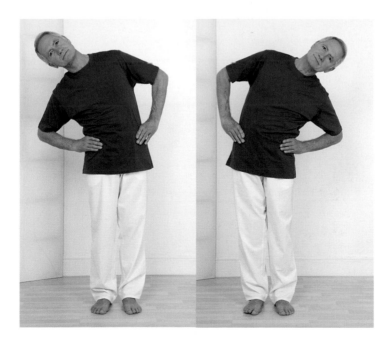

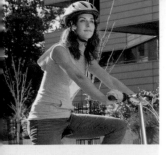

Carpal tunnel syndrome

BONES, JOINTS, AND MUSCLES

BEST MOVES

hand and wrist
exercises

walking

swimming

running

cycling

dancing

yoga

tai chi

Carpal tunnel syndrome is a sensation of pain, numbness, or tingling in your hand caused by pressure on the median nerve in your wrist. The median nerve and the nine tendons that bend your fingers run from the forearm to the hand through the carpal tunnel, which is located on the palm side of the wrist. The median nerve controls movement and feeling in the thumb and first three fingers, but not in the little finger.

Pressure on the median nerve can arise from swelling, or anything that reduces space in the carpal tunnel. Arthritis, diabetes, pregnancy, obesity, or repetitive wrist movements can contribute to the development of carpal tunnel syndrome. Sports involving prolonged use of the wrist and hand, such as tennis or golf, can give rise to the condition. Sometimes, just shaking your hand relieves symptoms.

Why exercise helps

People who are physically fit are generally at a lower risk for muscle, bone, and joint disorders. Those who do develop carpal tunnel syndrome may find that tai chi movements that relax the fingers, wrists, and forearms give some relief from symptoms. In addition, numerous exercises have been specifically designed to relieve pain and numbness in the wrists and hands, and restore normal use. "Gliding" exercises are most commonly used to help treat carpal tunnel syndrome (see pages 108–109). They relieve pressure on the median nerve and stretch the carpal ligaments. They also decrease the amount of fluid pressure in the hand and wrist by increasing blood flow out of the carpal tunnel. Research on the benefits of these exercises has had mixed results. People with mild to moderate carpal tunnel syndrome seem to benefit the most but severe cases may require surgery.

HOW OFTEN?

- Aerobic exercise for a minimum of 30 minutes 3–5 times per week is helpful.
- Practice yoga or tai chi at least once a week.
- Do gliding exercises and simple yoga hand/arm poses 3–5 times per day.

Opposite: *If you are putting in long hours on the bike, keep a light grip on the handle bars in order to avoid pressure on your wrists.*

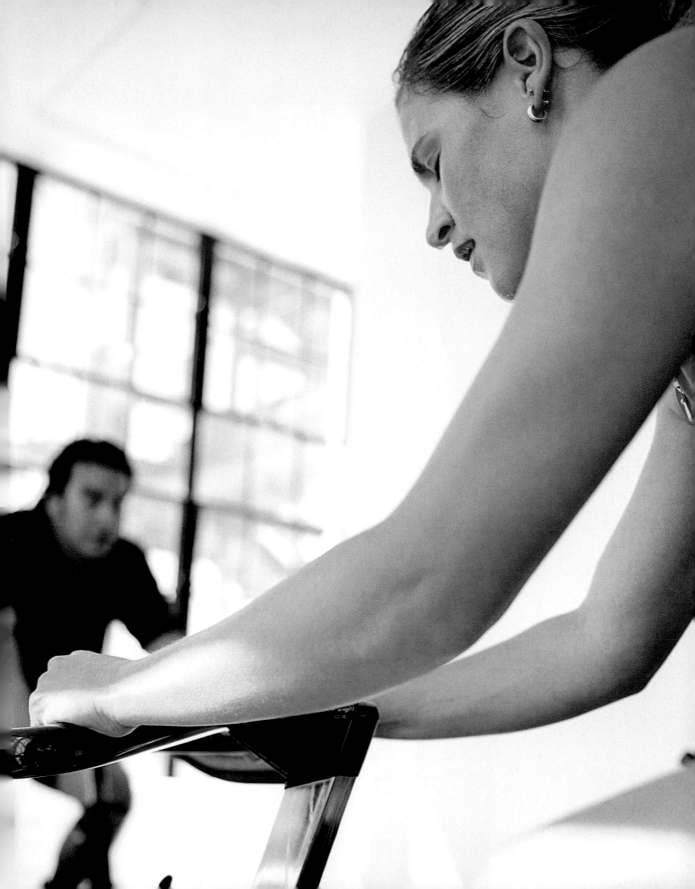

Exercises to help carpal tunnel syndrome

MEDIAN GLIDING EXERCISES *Hold each position for 7 seconds before moving on to the next, doing 5 repetitions of each.*

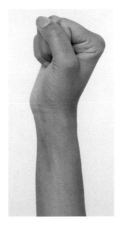 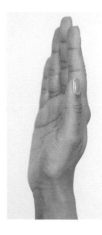 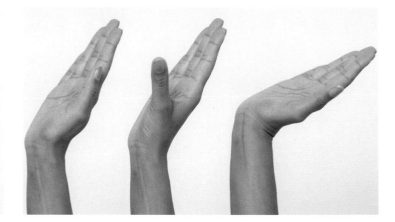

1. *Begin by making a fist and keeping your wrist in a neutral position.*

2. *Straighten and stretch your fingers and thumb.*

3. *Bend your wrist back, moving your thumb away from your palm.*

4. *Keep your palm facing upward and use your opposite hand to pull your thumb farther away from the palm.*

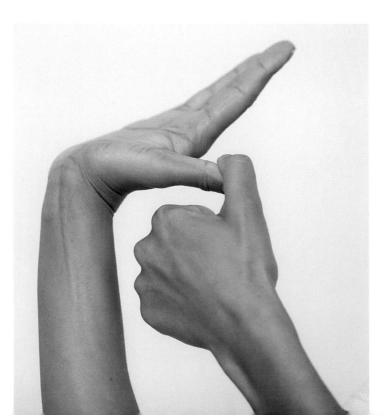

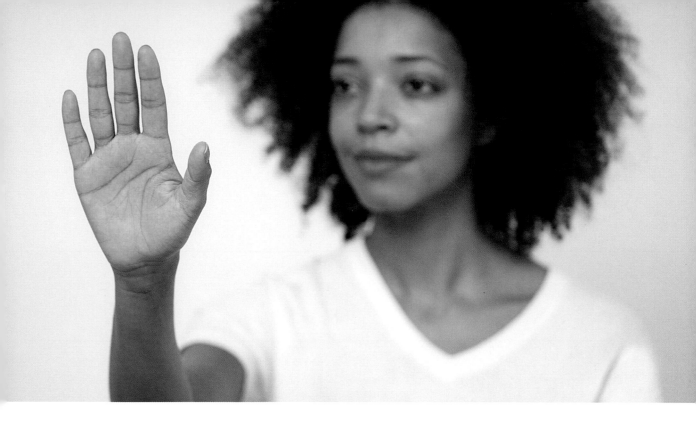

TENDON GLIDING EXERCISES *Hold each position for 7 seconds and do 10 repetitions.*

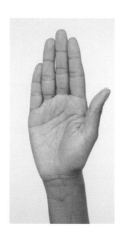 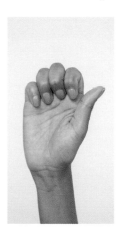 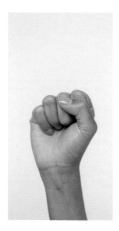 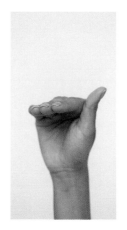 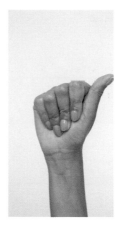

1. *Begin with your fingers straight.*

2. *Make a hook fist. Then return your fingers to the straight-hand position.*

3. *Next make a straight fist and then return your hand, once again, to the straight-hand position.*

4. *Bend the fingers at the knuckles with the thumb extending upward, then return to the straight-hand position.*

5. *Press the fingers lightly onto the palm, with thumb extended upward. Return to the straight-hand position.*

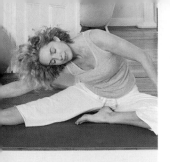

Chronic fatigue syndrome

BEST MOVES

walking

stretching

yoga

qigong

tai chi

light weight training

Feldenkrais

Chronic fatigue syndrome (CFS) is a disorder characterized by extreme and prolonged physical and mental exhaustion, which does not improve with rest. It is also sometimes known as myalgic encephalomyelitis (ME). In addition to fatigue, people with CFS often have a sore throat, aching lymph nodes in the neck or armpits, unexplained muscle and joint pain, headaches, and difficulties with memory and concentration. Although there are many theories about what causes this puzzling condition, including low blood pressure, depression, and viral infections, in most cases the cause cannot be established and symptoms can be difficult to measure.

Nevertheless, effective treatments for CFS exist and it is possible to recover from this frustrating and debilitating condition.

Why exercise helps

Exercise is difficult for people with CFS because they frequently lack the energy for physical exertion. Medical opinion has been divided on whether sufferers should attempt regular exercise or not—some believe that gentle exercise is helpful, while others caution against any form of aerobic activity. However, the sedentary lifestyle that is typical for most people with CFS leads to further health problems, including muscle wastage, loss of bone mass, and increased risk of obesity and cardiovascular disease. On balance, some exercise is better than none and may prove to be the road to recovery. Light exercise and stretching is not likely to worsen outcomes and can improve symptoms in many cases, leading to an increase in stamina and elevation of mood. People with CFS may find relief through the Feldenkrais method of exercise (see page 213), which is a slow, relaxing way of working with body movement.

Opposite: *Tai chi is slow and gentle but if it tires you, visualize the moves instead. Both tai chi and qigong can help raise the spirits, especially if performed outside.*

BONES, JOINTS, AND MUSCLES

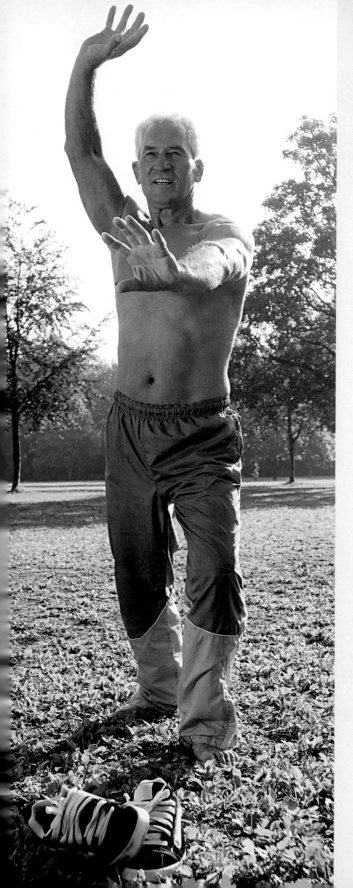

HOW OFTEN?

- Take an undemanding approach to physical activity, increasing the duration and intensity of exercise sessions very slowly. For example, if you can exercise for 5 minutes without suffering a relapse, try doing it for 6 minutes.

- Try one or two simple yoga poses and pay close attention to how they make you feel. If they don't exacerbate your symptoms, slowly add more. By undertaking short bursts of light exercise with long periods of rest in between, you may find you are able to do more without triggering exhaustion.

- Aerobic exercise is too taxing for many people with CFS. Attempt to walk for short distances, but if this is too much for you, stick with non-aerobic forms of exercise, such as stretching, gentle yoga, and weight training with light weights. Aim for a maximum of 3 exercise sessions per week. Experiment with what works for you and keep adjusting your program so that you are able to continue to exercise. It is counterproductive to try to push through the exhaustion. If walking for 15 minutes is not possible, walk for 5 minutes instead.

- If tai chi is too tiring, try qigong. Qigong can be performed with very little exertion without losing the benefit of its breathing techniques.

- Pacing yourself is very important. For example, you may find it easier to do stretches while lying down in bed and to focus on yoga poses that are done while lying down or sitting. Your goal should be to maintain a moderate level of daily activity, so that you are able to increase your stamina over time.

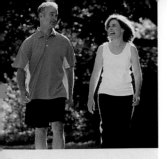

Fibromyalgia

BEST MOVES

walking

yoga

qigong

tai chi

slow dancing

Feldenkrais

stationary cycle

light weights

Pilates

BONES, JOINTS, AND MUSCLES

People suffering from fibromyalgia experience chronic intense pain in their muscles, connective tissues, and joints, and multiple tender points on the body where even slight pressure is painful. They also tend to have problems with concentration and memory. This debilitating syndrome causes fatigue, and associated anxiety and depression. Symptoms vary widely from person to person as does their intensity.

Fibromyalgia and chronic fatigue syndrome have many similarities, but the most prevalent symptom of fibromyalgia is widespread pain. Women are more likely to develop it than are men, and the risk increases with age.

Fibromyalgia symptoms can appear following mental or physical trauma, but in most cases there is no obvious cause. Recent research suggests that disorders in the central nervous system's pain-processing pathways are responsible, since people with fibromyalgia experience pain in response to stimuli that would not hurt anyone who is healthy. Relatively low levels of the mood-elevating chemical serotonin have been noted in sufferers, and impaired sleep phases.

There is no cure for fibromyalgia. A variety of prescription medications are often used to reduce pain levels and improve sleep. Rest and relaxation, stress reduction, a healthy diet, and gentle exercise are all necessary factors in helping to manage the syndrome successfully.

Why exercise helps

Aerobic exercise, strength training, and mind-body disciplines, such as yoga, qigong, and tai chi, are all helpful in treating fibromyalgia symptoms. They increase stamina and improve wellbeing. Regular exercise increases the body's production of endorphins, chemicals that boost mood and decrease pain. Studies have shown that people with fibromyalgia often find warm-water exercise beneficial. Exercise in heated water has improved pain thresholds, encouraged relaxation, reduced daytime fatigue, and resulted in improvements to cardiovascular capacity. However, those with a low tolerance for cold will need to exercise in a water temperature of around 90°F (32°C), which is several degrees warmer than most public heated pools.

Feldenkrais exercises (see page 213) are helpful for learning how to move in a way that lessens pain and improves breathing. Check whether a Feldenkrais Awareness Through Movement class is available near you. Otherwise, the Feldenkrais Lesson-a-Month archive online at www.flowingbody.com has instructions for slow, stretching exercises that you can do.

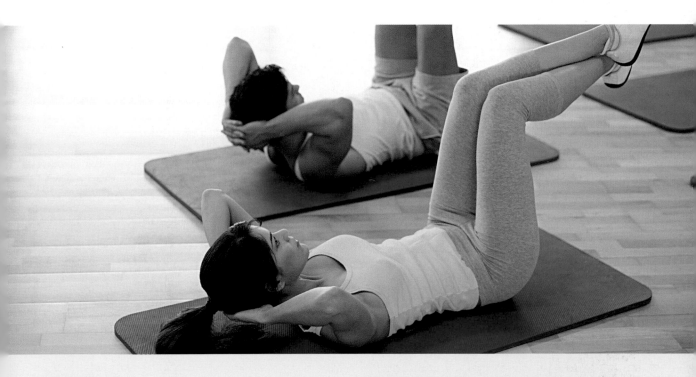

HOW OFTEN?

- Whichever form of exercise you choose, start slowly, with short, low-intensity sessions, and lengthen your workouts gradually, or add a second short session to your day. Keep a log of your progress—it will help you to be more engaged with your routine. Many people with fibromyalgia are prone to dizziness, so it may be wise to choose exercises or yoga poses for which you lie on the floor, sit down, or stand in a stable position.
- Begin with two sessions a week, several days apart, to assess how your body responds to the exercise. Know your limitations and stay within them. If you find a class is tiring you, slow down. Stop if necessary, even if the class hasn't finished. Don't exercise on a day when you are planning to undertake any other strenuous activity.
- Aim to do aerobic exercises for 20 minutes per day (split into two equal sessions, if you prefer) up to 3 times a week. Build up to this gradually, starting with 5 minutes on a stationary cycle, for example, and increasing this by 30 seconds or one minute each session.
- Build up to do strength training 3 times a week with 8–12 repetitions on an exercise machine or with light weights.

Above: *Low-impact Pilates is an ideal way to alleviate fibromyalgia pain.*

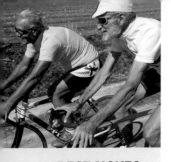

Lupus

BEST MOVES

walking

swimming

cycling

low-impact
aerobics

aqua aerobics

gentle yoga

tai chi

Pilates

stretching

elliptical/step
machines

Lupus, or systemic lupus erythematosus (SLE), is a complex disorder in which the immune system attacks healthy cells and tissues with resulting damage to joints, skin, blood vessels, and organs, in particular the heart, kidneys, and nervous system. Lupus can take many different forms, but common symptoms are intense joint pain or swelling, muscle pain, extreme fatigue, fever, and rashes. According to a recent study by the University of Trieste in Italy, 93 percent of people with lupus also suffer from anxiety and depression.

The cause of lupus is not known, but the fact that women of child-bearing age are more susceptible to it than men has suggested to researchers that the disease may be triggered by hormones such as estrogen. Symptoms tend to flare before menstrual periods or during pregnancy. The course of the disease is unpredictable, with phases of illness alternating with remission. There is no cure for lupus and it can be incapacitating, but medication and lifestyle changes can help to control it and some determined athletes that have been diagnosed with lupus have found that it is possible to continue training during remission.

Why exercise helps

As many as 80 percent of people with lupus experience fatigue, which may feel like an insurmountable barrier to taking exercise, but most people with the condition will benefit from some form of physical activity. Too much immobility weakens your muscles and prolongs feelings of exhaustion. Exercise, on the other hand, alleviates muscle stiffness, increases range of motion, and keeps the heart healthy. It strengthens bones and tones muscles without aggravating inflamed joints, while also helping to reduce the risk of osteoporosis.

Avoid activities that are hard on joints and muscles, such as running, weightlifting, or high-impact aerobics. Switch to non-weight-bearing exercise, such as cycling, swimming, or aqua aerobics. Cycling on a stationary bike or water exercise can also be very helpful if you are overweight and have a tendency to get joint pain or back pain when you exercise.

Two-thirds of people with lupus have increased sensitivity to light. If you are photosensitive, choose physical activities that you can do indoors, or cover up by wearing a hat, long-sleeved shirt, and long pants, and use a sunscreen if you walk or cycle outdoors.

Opposite: *For people with lupus, swimming is easy on the joints.*

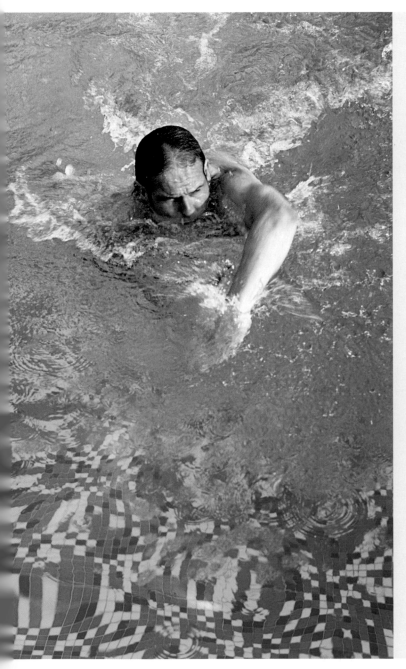

HOW OFTEN?

- Set a goal of 30 minutes on 3–5 days per week, but start slowly with a short session of 5–10 minutes to assess how much exertion you are able to tolerate.
- Try exercising early in the day, before you are too tired. You might begin with a 5–10-minute walk 3 times a week. Pace yourself, and gradually build up the duration and intensity of the exercise by 10 percent per week. For example, if you walk for 10 minutes, the next week add another minute per session.
- You could also consider exercising in short bursts several times a day. If you take a yoga, tai chi, or Pilates class, make sure you explain to the instructor that you have lupus and don't put pressure on yourself to keep up with what other people in the class are doing.
- Try not to give up exercising, because muscles that are not used will quickly atrophy. If you can afford it, hire a treadmill or stationary bicycle to use at home (working up to 30 minutes 3 times per week), so that exercise is more accessible and you don't have to deal with exposure to sunlight.
- Don't exercise if your joints feel hot, swollen, or tender, because exercise will make these symptoms worse.

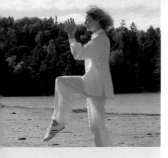

Neck pain

Neck pain is typically caused by prolonged poor posture, pinched nerves, or age-related wear and tear, such as osteoarthritis of the neck joints, or degeneration of the cervical spine. Engaging in repetitive tasks, such as working at a computer, frequently leads to persistent neck pain and this is caused by constriction in the trapezius muscle, which extends along the back of the neck. The most common form of neck pain arising from injury is the whiplash suffered in rear-end car collisions.

A combination of rest, medication, and therapeutic exercise usually relieves neck pain, though with varying degrees of success. If the pain persists, and becomes a chronic condition, your doctor may recommend that you undergo a rehabilitation course of physical therapy. Stretching and strength training are most beneficial for neck pain both as therapies and as preventive measures.

Why exercise helps

An ongoing Danish survey aimed at reducing repetitive strain injury has shown that neck muscle pain can be relieved by strength training using dumbbells. Stretching reduces pain and stiffness, and is a helpful therapy for people who have arthritis in the cervical joints. The sustained stretches offered by yoga and Pilates are ideal for strengthening, elongating, and relaxing muscles in the neck and back, and correcting postural misalignment. They can also relieve pressure on nerves or disks in the neck. Qigong's slow, meditative movements have been shown to alleviate chronic neck pain and shoulder and upper body tension. Qigong, like yoga, encourages deep breathing to calm the nervous system and to deliver more oxygen to the blood. Then gentle stretching directs an increase of nutrient-rich, oxygenated blood to the area of tension, and toxins are carried away, leaving the tight area more relaxed.

Opposite: *Neck muscle pain arising from repetitive strain injury can be relieved by strength training.*

BONES, JOINTS, AND MUSCLES

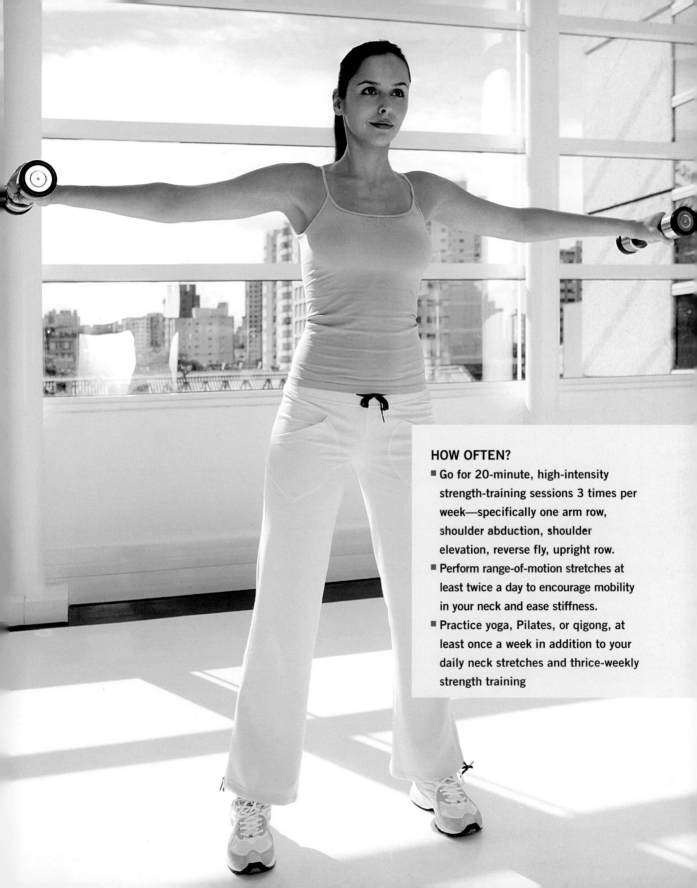

HOW OFTEN?
- Go for 20-minute, high-intensity strength-training sessions 3 times per week—specifically one arm row, shoulder abduction, shoulder elevation, reverse fly, upright row.
- Perform range-of-motion stretches at least twice a day to encourage mobility in your neck and ease stiffness.
- Practice yoga, Pilates, or qigong, at least once a week in addition to your daily neck stretches and thrice-weekly strength training

Five therapeutic yoga poses for the neck and upper back

GENTLE TWIST

1. *Sit facing forward with palms on the floor and a straight back. Keep your abdominal muscles strong.*

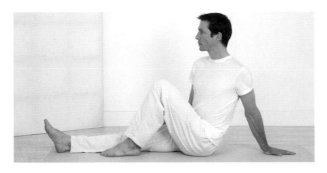

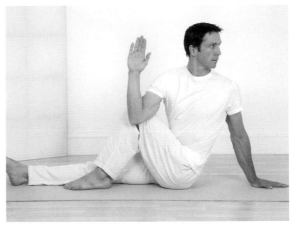

2. *Bend your left leg and press the palm of your left hand into the floor to help maintain an upright torso.*

3. *Turn your upper body and hook your right elbow over your left knee, with your palm outward as shown, to create a deep stretch in the thigh and lower back. Look along the line of your left shoulder, keeping your neck and shoulders relaxed. Repeat on the other side.*

TRIANGLE POSE

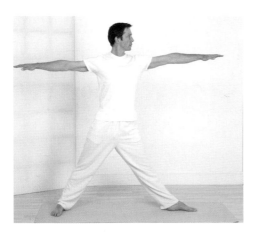

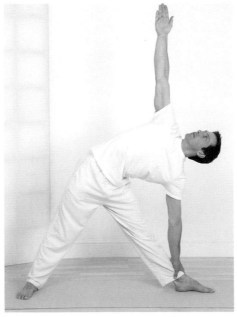

2. *Inhale then exhale as you lean to the left, holding your left ankle with a straight arm and aligning your right arm to create a vertical line. Look up to your right arm. Repeat on the other side.*

1. *Stand strong with your feet apart and arms extended, palms downward. Lift your pelvis and make sure your back is straight. Your toes should be at about the level of your wrists. Turn your left foot out.*

CAT POSE

1. Position yourself on all fours so your hands are aligned under your shoulders and your knees are in line with your hips.

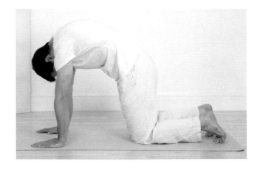

2. Tuck in your pelvis and lift your back, letting all tension go from your neck. Look down and let your neck relax and your head drop toward the floor.

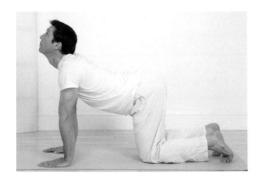

3. Now look up, arching your back and exhale. Repeat the rounding and arching of your back in a smooth rhythm for up to a minute, and then take Child's Pose and relax.

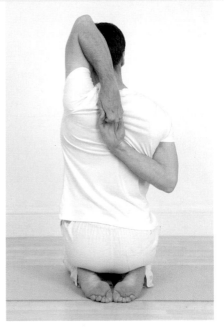

SHOULDER STRETCH

Sit in a kneeling position. Extend your left arm, then bend it behind your back to meet your bent right arm. Interlace your fingers. Breathe steadily as you feel the stretch over your shoulders. Keep your neck relaxed. Repeat on the other side. If your hands can't touch, use a strap.

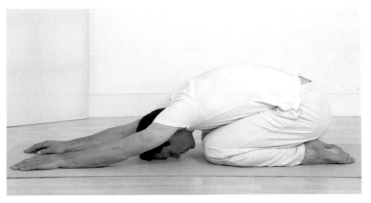

CHILD'S POSE

From a kneeling position, lean forward and place your forehead on the floor. Stretch your arms out in front and rest your palms and forearms on the floor. Breathe into the stretch.

Easy stretches to encourage ease of movement in the neck

Performed regularly, these stretches prevent the muscles in your neck from shortening and tightening. Do them slowly to the point where your muscles feel the stretch. Do not stretch to the point of pain. Breathing deeply, hold each stretch for 5 seconds. Repeat each stretch 5 times.

FLEXION

Bend head and neck forward with the aim of resting your chin on your chest. This elongates the muscles at the base of the cervical spine. You can experience a more intense stretch if you begin by tucking in your head and then bend your chin toward your chest. This is a wonderful stretch for countering the overly forward posture we develop from sitting at computers and driving cars.

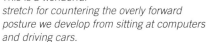

EXTENSION 1

Extend head and neck backward and look toward the ceiling. Make the movement smooth and slow in order not to crowd the small joints at the back of your neck.

EXTENSION 2

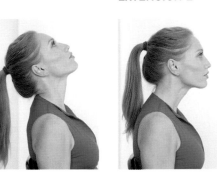

Extend head and neck forward, slowly and smoothly.

SIDE FLEXION

Bend ear down to shoulder. Try to keep your head from rotating when you do this stretch. This exercise stretches the neck area below the ears as well as the top of the shoulder.

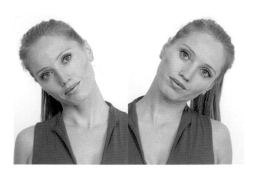

ROTATION

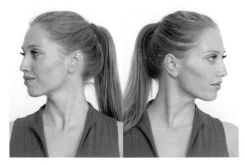

Turn head and neck from one side to the other, pausing at the end of each rotation to hold the stretch.

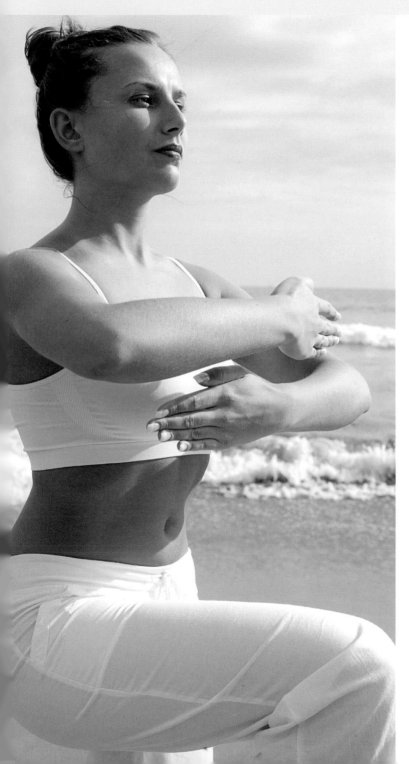

SHOULDER SHRUGS

Shrug your shoulders up and down in an exaggerated way. This helps to loosen up the shoulder area.

SHOULDER PRESSES

Press your shoulders to the front as if you were trying to get them to meet at the middle. Then press them right back, pulling your shoulder blades together.

QIGONG

There are many different types of gentle qigong exercises that relieve pain, stiffness, and tension in the neck and upper back. They often have fanciful names, such as "The Wise Owl Goes Backward" or "Rooster Spreads Feathers," but they are simple to perform. You can teach yourself qigong from a DVD and experiment with which exercises are most helpful for your neck pain, although the ideal is to attend a class and learn from a qualified qigong instructor.

Qigong is a healing discipline for the mind, body, and spirit. A workout lasting from 10 minutes to one hour consists of dynamic but gentle exercises, self-massage and, sometimes, meditation.

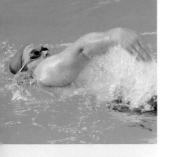

Sciatica

BEST MOVES
stretching
remedial yoga
Iyengar yoga
aqua exercise
walking
swimming
Feldenkrais

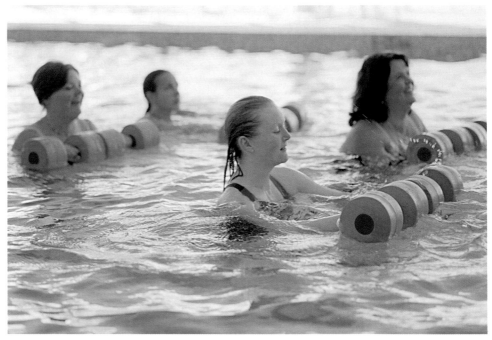

Sciatica is a term used to describe a set of painful symptoms caused by compression or irritation of the roots of the sciatic nerve at the base of the spine. Pain may begin abruptly or gradually anywhere along the route of the sciatic nerve running from the buttock down the back of the thigh into the calf and foot. It ranges from sharp pain through the lower back to a stabbing sensation in the buttock, or numbness or tingling, like an electric shock, that can radiate the entire length of the nerve.

The usual causes of sciatica are a lumbar spine disorder, such as a herniated (slipped) disk in the lower

Walking or running on the spot in warm water relieves the pain of sciatica.

back, spinal stenosis, which is narrowing of the spinal canal, and Piriformis Syndrome. The piriformis muscle is situated deep in the buttock and lies right on top of the sciatic nerve where it exits the spine. When the piriformis is tight, it puts pressure on the sciatic nerve, causing a sharp pain in the buttock and making walking and squatting difficult. Sciatic pain can also develop from general wear and tear on the lower spine. People with sciatica were once prescribed bed rest, but recent research has shown that the pain is more likely to be eased if you remain mobile and undertake careful exercise to recondition your lower back.

Why exercise helps

People experience the pain of sciatica in substantially different ways and it can require patience to find the exercises that are most beneficial for your condition and learn how to perform them correctly. You will need an accurate diagnosis, because the back exercises you do will vary according to the source of the pain. Consult with a physiotherapist or an instructor in remedial yoga to find what works for you. An experienced teacher of Iyengar yoga can show you how to use props to modify poses for your spine.

Certainly some physical activity is better than none. If you don't mobilize your back through gentle stretches and strengthening exercises, its muscles will weaken and make your sciatica worse. Back exercises are also important because movement encourages the exchange of nutrients and fluids within the spinal disks to keep them healthy.

Exercises to ease sciatica focus on strengthening the abdominal and back muscles in order to provide more support for the back, and on relaxing specific muscles, including the

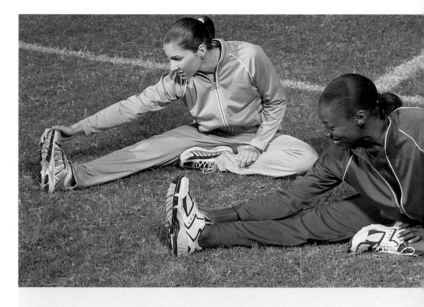

HOW OFTEN?
- Therapeutic stretching should be done twice daily.
- Walk for 15–30 minutes at least 3 times a week.
- Practice gentle yoga/aqua exercise for 30 minutes twice weekly.

piriformis, which have become inflexible. In general, walking is an excellent form of exercise for the lower back because it is relatively low impact but can provide all the benefits of an aerobic workout. A regular program of gentle aerobic exercise and stretching, especially stretching the hamstrings, will insure that your back remains healthy. If regular exercises are too painful for you to contemplate, aquatic exercises, or simply walking or running on the spot in the water, offer a relatively easy option.

Above: *Sciatica is often felt on one side only. If the pain radiates from the lower back, bring the leg in toward the groin on the side that is unaffected. If pain is focused in the buttocks, bend the painful leg. If pain persists, avoid seated forward bends.*

123

Gentle stretches for back health

The hamstrings are muscles located in the back of the thigh, running from the base of the buttocks to the knee. They help bend the knee and extend the hip. Tight hamstrings can cause a range of lower-back problems. Stretching them regularly can help to prevent sciatica.

SUPINE HAMSTRING STRETCH

A supine hamstring stretch, for which you lie on your back, is less stressful than a standing stretch for people who have had lower-back issues.

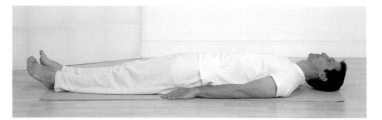

1. Lie on your back with a strap or towel to hand. Keep your abdominal muscles strong. Look up to the ceiling.

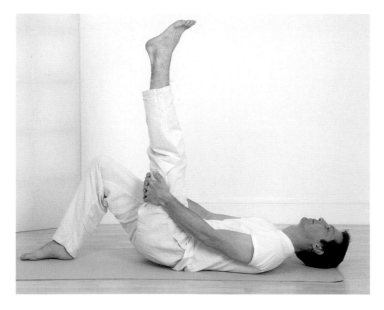

2. Bend both knees and clasp your hands around the back of one thigh, or support the thigh with the strap or towel. Slowly straighten the leg until you feel a stretch in the back of the thigh. Keep the other leg bent. Don't let your lower back arch or your hips move off the floor. Your aim is eventually to straighten the leg to a 90 degree angle, but don't force it. Hold the stretch for 10 seconds. Lower the leg to its original bent position and then stretch the other leg for 10 seconds. Repeat the stretch on both legs.

TIPS

■ People managing sciatica caused by a herniated disk should avoid rounding the back and avoid all seated forward bends; nor should they bend forward past 90 degrees with straight knees.

■ People managing sciatica caused by spinal stenosis benefit from forward bending and spine extensions. Flexing the lower spine—for example, lying on the back and pulling the knees to the chest—enlarges the spinal canal and relieves the impingement that is causing pain.

STRETCHING THE PIRIFORMIS MUSCLE

Stretching the piriformis muscle a few times a day, especially when combined with hamstring stretches, will prevent tightening of the lower back and relieve tension from hip to foot.

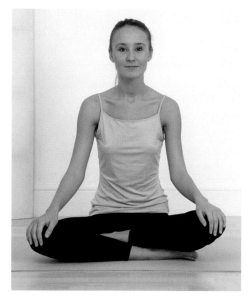

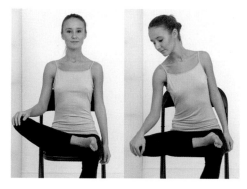

Sitting cross-legged: *One of the easiest ways to keep your hips open and stretch your piriformis muscle is by sitting cross-legged on the floor for several minutes a day.*

Chair stretch: *Another easy way to stretch out the piriformis, especially if you have a desk job, is to cross one leg over the other with your ankle resting on the knee of the opposite leg. Gently press down on the inside of the knee and slowly lean forward until you feel a mild stretch in the hips.*

Supine stretch: *Lie on your back with your legs stretched out. Pull one leg up toward your chest, holding the knee with the hand on the same side of the body. With the other hand, cautiously pull the knee across the body until you feel a stretch. Hold for 30 seconds. Repeat 3 times on each side.*

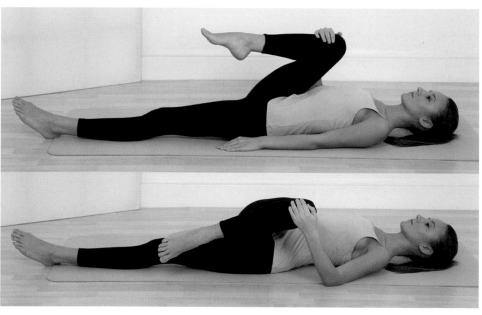

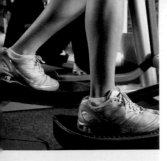

BEST MOVES

running

skipping

stair climbing

dancing

hiking

volleyball

tennis

basketball

power yoga

aqua aerobics

elliptical trainer

Osteoporosis

Osteoporosis means literally "porous bone." When osteoporosis occurs, the "holes" in the bones' spongy tissue increase in number and expand in size, making bones fragile and more likely to break. Although osteoporosis occurs in both men and women, women are four times as likely to develop the disease as are men, and are particularly susceptible after menopause, when bones lose density and strength.

Often osteoporosis progresses without any symptoms or pain until a fragility fracture occurs, most often in the hip, spine, or wrist. However, a healthy diet and regular weight-bearing exercise (activities you do on your feet with your bones supporting your weight) can slow the rate of bone loss or prevent osteoporosis from occurring.

Why exercise helps

Bones need to be stressed in order to become stronger. The "pounding" of high-impact, dynamic, endurance activities, especially running, is very effective for developing bone-mineral density. Playing basketball, tennis, or volleyball is also a good option.

A comparative study by the University of Missouri showed that running builds stronger spines than non-weight-bearing activities, such as cycling, swimming, or rowing. Researchers in Sweden studying older men and the link between osteoporosis and exercise found that one-third of fractures could be prevented if men could be persuaded to take part in sports regularly. For maximum bone health, add running or another high-impact activity to your exercise regimen. Vigorous forms of yoga that require jumps and weight-bearing push-ups in between poses, such as ashtanga and others with vinyasa flow (where poses run together with synchronized breathing and movement), are also helpful for strengthening bones.

If running and other high-impact activity are too much for you, walk instead. Walking is an effective weight-bearing exercise and it minimizes jarring to your bones. Aqua aerobics also has minimal impact on bones and joints. Dancing is excellent exercise for people with osteoporosis because it is a weight-bearing activity and it also increases flexibility, coordination, and balance. Thirty minutes of cha cha or samba provides the equivalent to a moderate-level aerobic workout.

If your ability to exercise is compromised by scoliosis or the pain of fibromyalgia, common conditions in women with osteoporosis, you may want to consider trying something less strenuous, such as yoga, qigong, or Pilates, or working out on an elliptical machine.

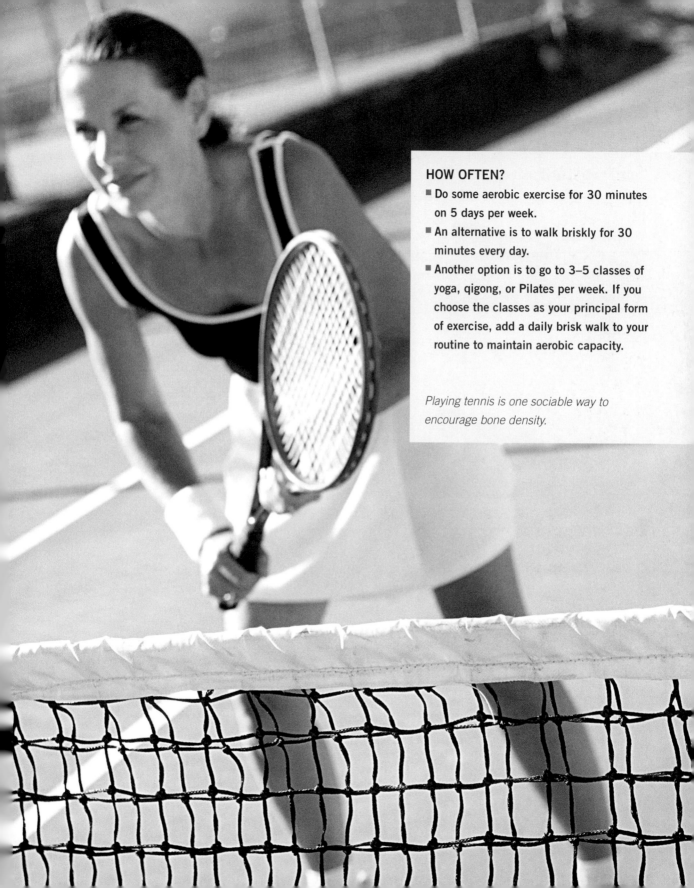

HOW OFTEN?

- Do some aerobic exercise for 30 minutes on 5 days per week.
- An alternative is to walk briskly for 30 minutes every day.
- Another option is to go to 3–5 classes of yoga, qigong, or Pilates per week. If you choose the classes as your principal form of exercise, add a daily brisk walk to your routine to maintain aerobic capacity.

Playing tennis is one sociable way to encourage bone density.

Weight-bearing exercises for strong bones

THE PLANK AND PUSH-UP

Aim: To work the core muscles and develop upper-body strength; to tone the arms.

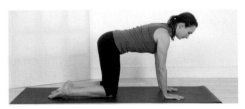

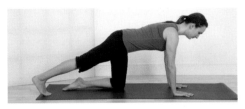

1. Kneel with hands beneath your shoulders, knees directly under your hips, and feet in line with the knees. Lengthen from the crown of your head to the tailbone, and keep the neck long. Draw in the stomach.

2. Breathe in, then breathe out, pull in the stomach, and slide the right leg directly behind you in line with the hip. Tuck the toes under.

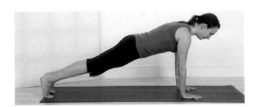

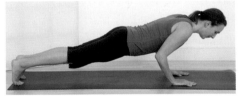

5. Breathe out to release the right foot and slide the leg back beneath the hip. Follow with the left leg until you are back in the starting position. Keep the pelvis still throughout.

3. Breathe in, breathe out, and follow with the left leg. Your back and pelvis stay still, in a straight line. Keep legs parallel and hip-width apart. The weight is evenly distributed between hands and feet.

4. Breathe in and slowly bend your elbows toward the waist. Dip just a little. Keep your neck long and eyes focused on the floor to prevent the head from dropping. Breathe out and slowly straighten the elbows. Repeat 5 times.

REACH EXERCISE (Table Top)

Aim: To strengthen core muscles and develop coordination and balance; to strengthen the upper body, particularly the arms and wrists; to work the gluteals.

1. Kneel as in the plank, position 1. Lengthen from the crown of your head to the tailbone, and keep the neck long. Breathe in to prepare.

2. Breathe out, draw the stomach in and slide one leg away, simultaneously sliding the opposite hand along the floor in line with the shoulder. Lengthen and lift the arm and leg no higher than your body. The pelvis must stay square with the floor.

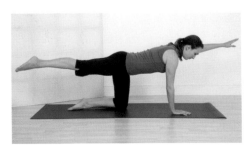

3. Breathe in to lower your arm and leg to the floor, and breathe out to slide your limbs back. Repeat up to 5 times on each side.

BALANCE

Aim: To center the body, challenging the balance, strengthening the ankles and feet; to open the shoulders.

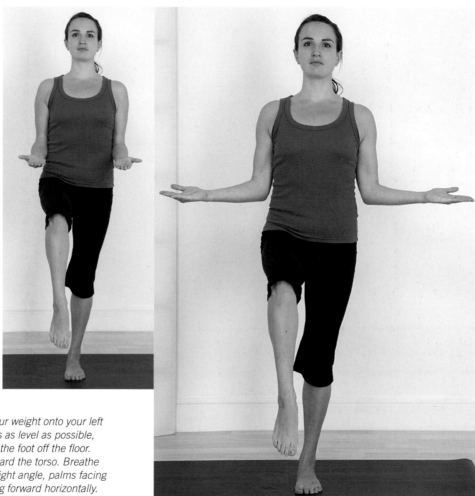

1. Stand tall on the floor and lengthen the spine. Legs are parallel and hip-width apart. Breathe in to prepare.

2. Breathe out, transfer your weight onto your left leg, and, keeping the pelvis as level as possible, bend your right knee to lift the foot off the floor. Draw the leg up and in toward the torso. Breathe in, bend your elbows to a right angle, palms facing up and forearm lengthening forward horizontally.

3. Breathe in and, keeping the elbows drawn in to the waist, turn your arms outward from the shoulder, reaching your forearms wide. Keep the stomach lifted. Breathe out as you return the arms to the start position, and the foot to the floor.

4. Lengthen through the spine, adjust the weight on the feet, and repeat on the other side. Repeat up to 8 times on each side.

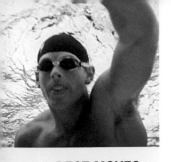

BEST MOVES

swimming

aqua exercise

strength training

stretching

stationary cycling

Iyengar yoga

remedial yoga

walking

Feldenkrais

exercise plus Alexander technique

Back pain

Back pain is responsible for more everyday functional disability than any other condition in Western societies. It is usually the result of strained muscles or ligaments caused by stressful movements, such as a sudden twisting motion or lifting a heavy object carelessly or awkwardly. Structural problems, including a ruptured disk (disks are the "cushions" between the spine's vertebrae), arthritis, sciatica, and scoliosis, also cause back pain. Acute pain caused by strains generally heals relatively quickly and can be treated variously with medications, heat/ice therapy, and rest. Chronic back pain—that is, pain lasting for more than two weeks—should be treated with appropriate stretching and strengthening exercises to ease symptoms.

Why exercise helps

Injections and medications can provide pain relief but they don't spur the healing process. Healing is stimulated by physical activity. Future episodes of back pain are less likely to occur if you follow a fitness routine that provides aerobic conditioning, exercises to strengthen your back, and stretches to relax tight muscles. When you exercise your back, nutrients are released into the back's soft tissues and the space around spinal disks, and they keep the muscles, ligaments, and joints healthy. Regular exercise also improves your awareness of body mechanics and so helps you to find ways to avoid injury.

Stretches alleviate muscle stiffness and increase range of motion. Hamstring stretching is important because tight hamstrings limit motion in the pelvis, which in turn can increase stress across the lower back. A healthy spine needs to be supported by a strong core, so you will need to exercise your abdominal muscles and gluteal muscles. As an intervention for back pain, strength training, using weights and other load-bearing exercise equipment, is more effective than jogging, walking on a treadmill, or using an elliptical machine. But it is important to be aerobically fit as well as strong. Water therapy, or aqua exercise, is a great way to get a benign aerobic workout. The water counteracts gravity and provides buoyancy as well as mild resistance. Continuous brisk walking, rather than stop-start walking, helps to build fitness, and cycling on a stationary bike provides aerobic conditioning with minimal impact on the spine. This is also a good exercise option for people who are more comfortable positioned leaning forward.

Exercise and the Alexander technique

An exercise program in combination with lessons in the Alexander technique offers long-term effective treatment for

Right: *Side muscles (obliques) help support the spine. Keep them strong and flexible with regular stretching.*

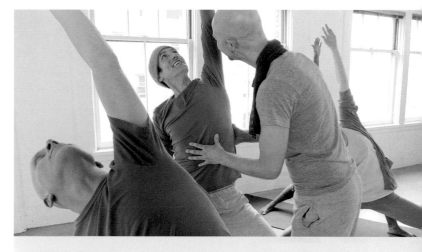

chronic back pain and improved quality of life, according to research from the universities of Southampton and Bristol.

The Alexander technique uses personalized training to develop skills that improve postural tone and muscular coordination. Over a course of sessions, your teacher helps you release muscular tension and you learn how to sit, stand, and move safely and easily.

Yoga

In a large, long-term study funded by the United States National Institutes of Health on the efficacy of yoga for healing chronic lower-back problems, researchers found that people who did Iyengar yoga overcame pain and depression more successfully than those who followed conventional treatments for lower-back pain. Iyengar yoga delivers strength, flexibility, and balance skills by emphasizing the precise alignment of the body in the various poses. The participants in the study who practiced yoga also reduced their use of pain medication more than a control group who received standard medical care.

HOW OFTEN?

- Prevent back pain by conditioning your body with 3–5 sessions of aerobic exercise and strength training per week. If you are out of shape, build up fitness by walking at a sustained pace for a minimum of 20–30 minutes per day 5 times per week, or exercise in a swimming pool for 30 minutes 3 times a week.
- People with chronic back pain may find that 5–10 minutes of stretching in the morning and at night can provide relief from lower-back pain.
- To strengthen the back muscles, 15–20 minutes of prescribed exercises should be done every other day. Strengthening exercises are best done on alternate days to allow the body to rest those muscles. Low-impact aerobics (such as walking, cycling, or swimming) should be done for 30–40 minutes 3 times weekly, on alternate days from the strengthening exercises.
- If you are focusing on yoga as a therapy, try to do a minimum of 2 classes per week with a qualified Iyengar teacher. It is essential to tell the instructor that you have chronic lower-back pain. You may also be able to find remedial yoga classes that target back pain.

131

Stretches for the back and legs

Do these stretches once or twice a day to take stress off the lower back and hips.

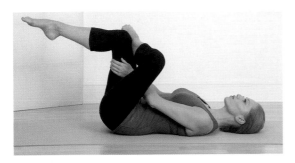

PIRIFORMIS STRETCH

The piriformis muscle runs from the back of the thigh bone to the sacrum at the base of the spine. Tightness in this muscle is linked to lower-back pain and sometimes pain along the sciatic nerve.

Lie on your back and bend your knees. Cross your right leg over your left thigh. Place both hands together under the knee of your left leg (the lower leg), and gently pull the leg toward your chest. Hold both thighs until a stretch is felt in the buttock area. Hold for 30 seconds. Repeat by crossing your left leg over the right leg.

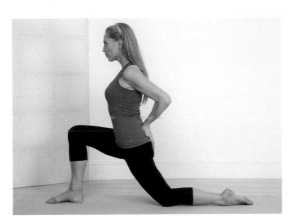

PSOAS MAJOR STRETCH

The psoas major muscle is attached to the front portion of the lower spine and can greatly limit lower-back mobility when tight.

Kneel on your right knee, left foot flat on the floor, left knee bent. Rotate the right leg outward. Place your hand on the right gluteus muscle and tighten the muscle. Lean forward through your hip, being careful not to bend the lower spine. You should feel the stretch in the front of your right hip. Hold for 30 seconds. Repeat on the other side.

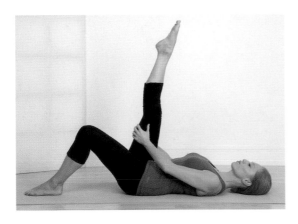

HAMSTRING STRETCH

The hamstrings run from the back of the pelvic bone to just below the back of the knee. They are responsible for bending the knee and help the gluteal muscles to extend the hip. Tight hamstrings make it difficult to sit up straight and they are also associated with lower-back pain.

To stretch your hamstring muscles gently, lie on your back with both legs bent. Grasp one leg behind the knee and attempt to straighten it with the toes pointed back toward you. Hold for 30 seconds and repeat with the other leg.

Chapter 7

Digestive System

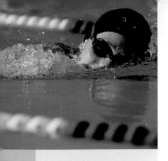

Constipation

DIGESTIVE SYSTEM

BEST MOVES

walking

jogging

running

hiking

cycling

swimming

rowing

dancing

capoeira

stretching

yoga

qigong

tai chi

Pilates

When ingested food moves too slowly through the gastrointestinal tract, the colon absorbs all of its water content, rendering it into dry, hard feces, which are difficult and painful to expel. If the feces remain in the bowel for three days or more, the digestive system becomes constipated and the incomplete defecation causes chronic abdominal pain. If left untreated, constipation can lead to irritable bowel syndrome. Severe constipation can also cause obstruction in the bowel with serious consequences.

Constipation can be caused by a low-fiber diet, by hemorrhoids or anal fissures, or by an overuse of laxatives. It is also a side effect of some medications and is quite common during pregnancy. A balanced diet, with plenty of fiber and fluid intake, and regular exercise are recommended for the relief of constipation.

Why exercise helps

Physical activity plays a key role in the prevention and management of constipation. Aerobic exercise accelerates breathing and heart rate, which helps to stimulate intestinal contractions and digestive enzymes. Efficient contractions speed up the amount of time that ingested food takes to travel through the large intestine. However, wait for at least an hour after a large meal before engaging in strenuous exercise. Blood flow in the stomach and intestines increases after you've eaten in order to digest the food. If you exercise too soon after a meal, the blood is diverted toward the heart and the limbs, which undermines the digestive action in the gastrointestinal tract, making it sluggish and more likely to produce excess gas and cramps.

Stretching can also help alleviate constipation, as can certain yoga poses and qigong and tai chi moves. Yoga poses helpful for relieving constipation are backward bends, such as Cobra and Bow, and the Half Spinal Twist. Inverted poses, such as Headstand and Shoulder Stand, are particularly helpful for constipation, since they give the large intestines some relief from gravitational compression.

Opposite: *Exercise relieves constipation by decreasing the time it takes for food to travel through the intestine.*

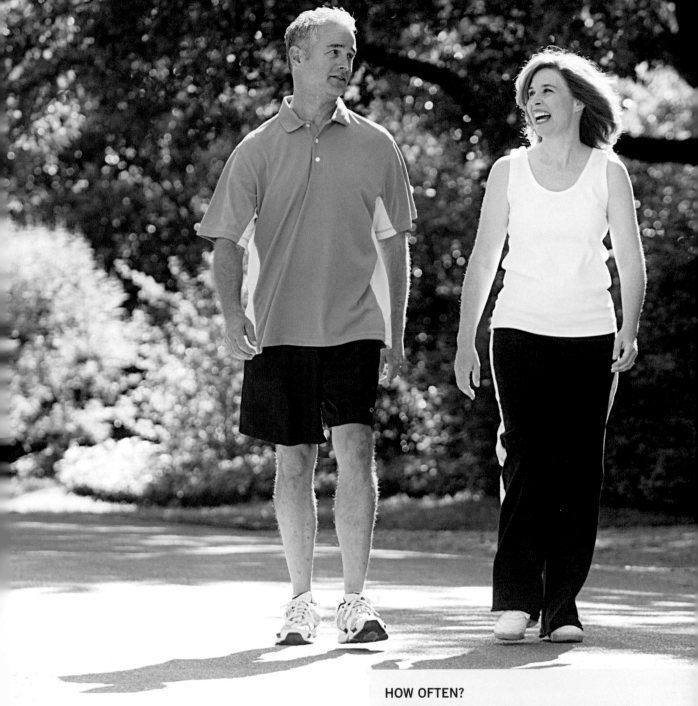

HOW OFTEN?

■ Walking for 10–15 minutes several times a day can help your body to digest food more efficiently than it would otherwise. Take more vigorous exercise for 30 minutes 5 times a week.

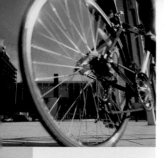

BEST MOVES

walking

slow jogging

cycling

elliptical trainer

yoga

tai chi

qigong

Gastritis

Gastritis is inflammation of the stomach lining. It is most commonly caused by bacterial infection, which damages the mucus lining that normally protects the stomach from acidic digestive juices. Gastritis can also be caused by severe stress, excess stomach acid, or excessive use of alcohol or non-steroidal, anti-inflammatory drugs, or drugs that contain ibuprofen or aspirin. Symptoms, which can vary in intensity, are upper abdominal discomfort or pain, indigestion, heartburn, nausea, vomiting, and loss of appetite. When gastritis is severe a peptic ulcer may develop.

Why exercise helps

Any form of exercise that increases breathing and heart rate also helps to stimulate the activity of intestinal muscles and allows food waste to travel quickly through the colon. Regular exercise will improve overall health and immune response as well as helping the digestive system to become more efficient.

Breathing exercises and the mind-body practices of yoga, tai chi, and qigong promote relaxation and are helpful for reducing stress and the production of excess stomach acid. The physical up-and-down movements of the diaphragm encouraged by qigong also have a beneficial effect on the digestive system and alleviate gastric troubles, as do yoga poses such as Standing Forward Bend, Cobra, and Thunderbolt, which massage internal organs.

HOW OFTEN?

■ The intensity and duration of exercise will vary according to the severity of symptoms. Start slowly if you are concerned about triggering an attack of gastritis. If possible, aim for 30 minutes of aerobic exercise at least 3 times per week.

Opposite: *Aerobic exercise helps the digestive system to become more efficient and alleviates gastric discomfort.*

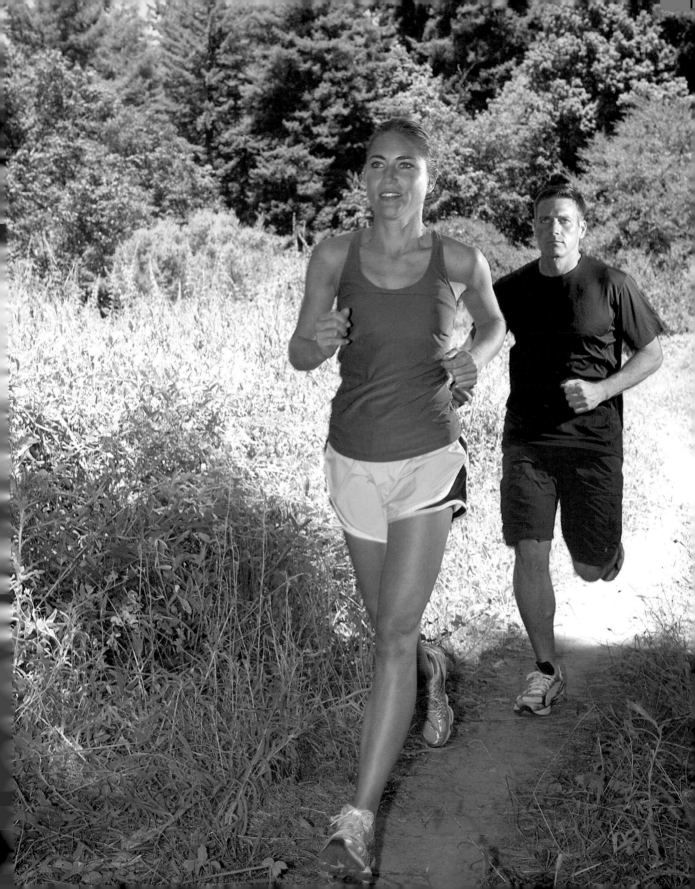

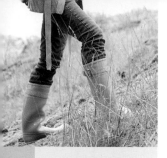

Heartburn and GERD

BEST MOVES

walking

cycling

spinning

hiking

tai chi

Nearly everyone experiences heartburn occasionally—a burning sensation in the chest that occurs after eating and is sometimes accompanied by a sour taste of stomach acid. Normally, the lower esophageal sphincter prevents digestive acid in the stomach from backing up into the esophagus, but pressure on the sphincter muscle from excess weight, overeating, or lying down too soon after a meal may cause it to open slightly and allow stomach contents to return to the esophagus, a process known as reflux. When the refluxed stomach acid touches the lining of the esophagus, a burning sensation is created in the chest or throat. Frequent, persistent heartburn may be a symptom of gastroesophageal reflux disorder (GERD)—the chronic regurgitation of stomach acid. People with GERD may have chest pain, trouble swallowing, bad breath, and a dry cough. Contributing factors for GERD include alcohol, obesity, pregnancy, and smoking. Eating citrus fruits, chocolate, fatty and fried foods, minty foods, garlic, onions, and spicy foods, and consuming caffeinated drinks, may trigger GERD.

THE FOLLOWING GUIDELINES WILL HELP TO ESTABLISH A COMFORTABLE REGIMEN

Carbs not fat: Before you work out, eat a meal high in carbohydrates and low in fat and protein (see below for timing). Avoid trigger foods, including chocolate, citrus fruit, caffeinated drinks, and any spicy or fatty foods.

Let your food digest: Wait at least two hours after meals before you start exercising. If you are planning to run, wait for three hours.

Don't dehydrate: Water helps the process of digestion, so make sure you drink plenty of it.

Lower the intensity: High-impact exercise jiggles the contents of your stomach and as a result can increase the likelihood of incurring acid reflux. Try some calmer activities, such as cycling, skating, or walking.

Stay upright: Some people get heartburn when they lie down, or bend over, so you may want to avoid exercises that require those positions—bench presses, certain yoga postures and Pilates moves, and swimming, for example. Instead, go for flowing, upright tai chi.

Medicine: Taking an antacid preparation an hour before exercising may help.

Chest pain: The pain of heartburn is similar to pain caused by heart problems. If you have chest pain, have it checked out by your doctor.

DIGESTIVE SYSTEM

Why exercise helps

Excess fat on the walls of the stomach can interfere with digestion. Regular exercise encourages weight loss, which decreases the chance of getting heartburn, and aids digestion by limiting the secretion of stomach acid. People who have developed GERD will also benefit from frequent, moderate exercise, which can reduce symptoms, increase fitness, and give a sense of wellbeing. Stress management reduces symptoms, too. For this, you may want to try tai chi, qigong, meditation, and deep-breathing techniques.

When it comes to more vigorous forms of exercise, some care needs to be taken. Many people find that their acid reflux symptoms are aggravated by intense, jarring activities, such as running, aerobics, and weightlifting, which increase pressure on the esophageal sphincter, making it more prone to open and admit stomach acid into the esophagus. Sit-ups, crunches, and other exercises that tense the stomach muscles may also be better avoided. However, responses to exercise can vary widely in people with GERD. You may have to experiment to find the exercises that are best for you.

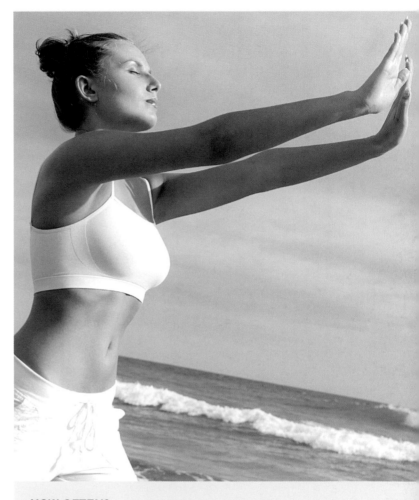

HOW OFTEN?

- Take moderate exercise for 30 minutes 3–5 days per week. If your symptoms are under control, try to do more.
- Practice qigong for at least 5 minutes per day and tai chi for 15–30 minutes at least 3 days per week.

Above: *If you suffer from heartburn, avoid exercise that involves jumping and jarring movements.*

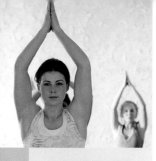

BEST MOVES

walking

cycling

swimming

yoga

Pilates

qigong

tai chi

Irritable bowel syndrome

People with irritable bowel syndrome (IBS) suffer from overactive nerves and muscles in the colon. IBS causes the muscular contractions that pass food along the gastrointestinal tract to be abnormally strong, which results in painful symptoms of cramping, bloating, gas, and either diarrhea or constipation, depending on what area of the gut is overactive. Triggers for IBS can range from medications to emotions to intestinal pressure after eating certain foods. It is not known why this sensitivity develops, although about half of people with IBS can link the onset of colon spasms to a stressful event. Symptoms tend to become worse during times of stress or anxiety. This is because the colon is partly controlled by the autonomic nervous system, which responds to stress.

Why exercise helps

Chronic ailments, such as IBS, are fatiguing. Regular physical activity will increase the amount of oxygen in your blood and raise energy levels. Exercise helps relieve depression and stress, and eases the abnormal contractions of the intestines. If you are new to exercise, start with gentle workouts, such as walking, slow cycling, swimming, yoga, qigong, tai chi, or Pilates mat work. Qigong, tai chi, and yoga will decrease anxiety and soothe the body's nervous system. Yoga's Legs Up The Wall pose (see page 73) relieves constipation. The Cobbler, or Butterfly, pose eases diarrhea (see page 73). Sit with your back straight, let your legs open, and place the soles of the feet together.

If you are reasonably fit, having IBS should not affect your ability to undertake most forms of exercise, although be aware that demanding activities, such as long-distance running, have been associated with triggering diarrhea symptoms. You can reduce the likelihood of getting runner's diarrhea by letting two hours pass between eating and exercising, and by avoiding caffeine and fatty or gas-producing foods. If you have diarrhea and are worried about exercising in a public place, buy a couple of exercise DVDs and devise a home-based routine for yourself.

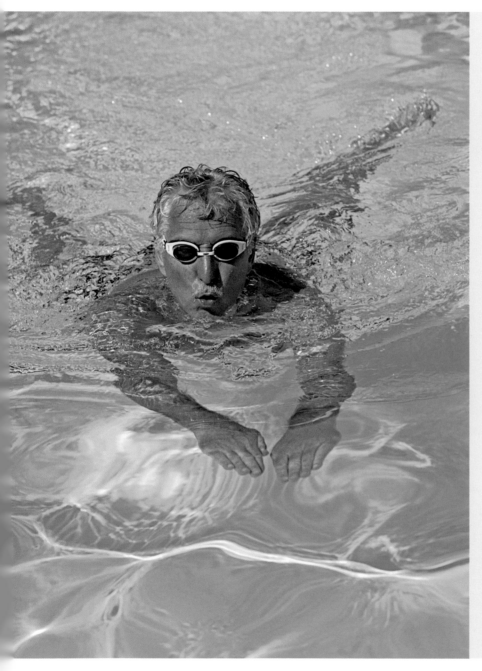

HOW OFTEN?

- If you've been inactive, start slowly and gradually increase the amount of time you exercise. Try to time your workouts so you exercise at the times when your intestines are quieter.
- Aim to walk daily for 10–20 minutes.
- Swim or cycle 3 times per week for 30 minutes each session.

Gentle swimming is calming and eases the stress of irritable bowel syndrome.

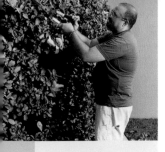

Hemorrhoids

BEST MOVES

walking

running

swimming

stair climbing

dancing

gardening

tennis

Pilates

yoga

tai chi

Hemorrhoids are dilated veins that develop in the area of the lower rectum. Internal hemorrhoids, which develop inside the rectum, usually remain small and subside relatively quickly, although they can cause bleeding during a bowel movement. External hemorrhoids protrude from the anus. They can be painful and cause itching or a burning sensation. People with chronic constipation or who habitually strain to move their bowels are susceptible to hemorrhoids. Many pregnant women develop hemorrhoids because the uterus compresses veins as it expands and obstructs the return of blood from the rectum.

DON'T STRAIN

If you have hemorrhoids, straining to have a bowel movement will enlarge them. Eating a high-fiber diet, drinking copious amounts of water, and undertaking regular exercise will help soften your stools and prevent irritation of the hemorrhoids.

To ease the expulsion process, try the following moves while you are sitting on the toilet

■ Sit up straight and lean back slightly.
■ Raise your arms above your head to stretch the colon. Move from side to side.
■ Contract and expand your abdomen to help move your colon.

Why exercise helps

Regular exercise prevents hemorrhoids forming because it activates blood flow, which encourages healthy functioning of the digestive system and helps to regulate bowel movements. If you have already developed hemorrhoids, exercise is an effective way of healing them but avoid activities that can aggravate rectal veins, such as lifting weights or cycling.

Sitting down for long periods will increase pressure on your hemorrhoids. An activity as basic as a daily walk around the block will help. Swimming is soothing and so are yoga poses that massage colon and anus muscles. Try jumping on a rebounder to oxygenate the blood and get lymph fluid moving (see page 175). If you are stuck in front of a desk for hours on end, get up and walk around for five minutes at least once an hour, or do some stair climbing in your office building.

DIGESTIVE SYSTEM

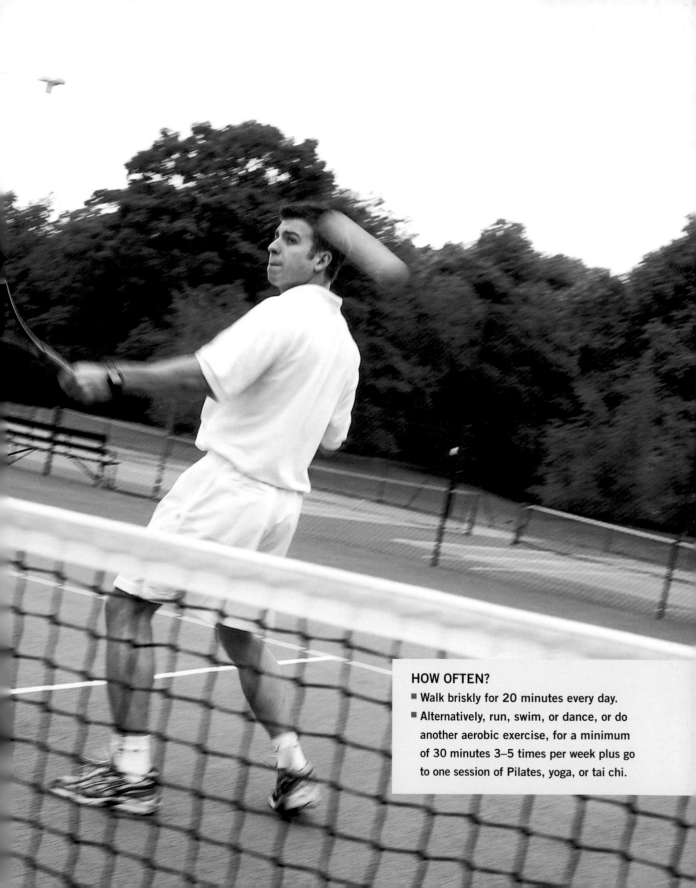

HOW OFTEN?
- Walk briskly for 20 minutes every day.
- Alternatively, run, swim, or dance, or do another aerobic exercise, for a minimum of 30 minutes 3–5 times per week plus go to one session of Pilates, yoga, or tai chi.

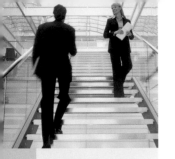

Inflammatory bowel disease

BEST MOVES

walking

jogging

swimming

stair climbing

circuit training

spinning

light
weight lifting

qigong

yoga

tai chi

Pilates

Inflammatory bowel disease (IBD) refers to the intestinal inflammation that is symptomatic of ulcerative colitis and Crohn's disease. Usually these conditions are treated with medication, exercise, and sometimes surgery. Ulcerative colitis inflames the linings of the colon and rectum. As a result, water cannot be absorbed into the bloodstream, which leads to chronic diarrhea, cramps, and rectal bleeding. Severe cases require hospitalization to manage diarrhea, blood loss, and the risk of malnutrition.

Crohn's disease can involve any part of the gastrointestinal tract, but most commonly affects the small intestine and/or the colon. The intestinal wall becomes swollen, inflamed, and ulcerated, causing abdominal pain, often in the lower right side, diarrhea, rectal bleeding, and fever. In severe cases, the intestine becomes blocked by swelling and scar tissue.

IBD occurs most frequently in the late teens and twenties. Its causes are unclear but it may be an autoimmune disorder in which the immune system mistakenly attacks the intestinal tract and other parts of the body. IBD tends to run in families, so there may be a genetic predisposition. There is little evidence that stress causes IBD, although stress may aggravate symptoms. IBD can flare up and then subside for a time, and the symptoms can vary from mild to severe.

People with IBD often suffer weight loss and fatigue, and around 30 percent are affected by arthritis, mainly when the disease is active.

Why exercise helps

There is no proof that exercise can prevent the onset of inflammatory bowel disease, but exercise can help reduce its

EXERCISE TIPS

- Avoid solid foods for three hours before aerobic exercise.
- Drink plenty of fluids.
- Avoid extreme changes in body temperature during exercise.
- Minimize impact. Try calm activities, such as swimming, yoga, tai chi, and Pilates. Yoga and Pilates are also excellent for strengthening the pelvic-floor muscles.
- Walk don't run, if you are worried about incontinence. On a treadmill, increase the track's elevation.
- Plan exercise activities so that you are near a bathroom, in case you should experience diarrhea or other bowel symptoms.
- Listen to your body and plan accordingly. If you feel a flare-up coming on, don't push yourself physically. It's important to strike a balance between rest and exercise.

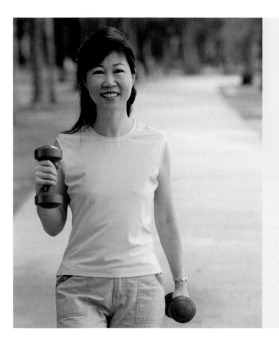

HOW OFTEN?

- Some people with IBD may be able to undertake limited amounts of exercise only, but even 10–15 minutes of walking per day, or a gentle yoga or qigong class once a week, will be of benefit.
- If you have IBD-related joint stiffness, you may find it easier to exercise later in the day when your joints have loosened up.
- If you feel quite well in between flare-ups, aim for 30-minute exercise sessions 3–5 times per week.

Exercise between flare-ups, when you have more energy and are feeling well. Intense exercise while going through an IBD attack may cause extreme fatigue.

symptoms. The drugs that keep IBD under control often cause lethargy and weight gain, and exercise helps to shed weight, increase energy levels, and improve a sense of wellbeing and immunological response. Exercise can also help to relieve the depression sometimes associated with IBD.

The type, intensity, and frequency of activity will depend on individual symptoms. If your symptoms are stable, you should be able to pursue most sport and fitness activities, even vigorous ones, such as running, kickboxing, or spinning classes. If you experience a flare-up of diarrhea or abdominal pain, back off from exercise and wait until you are feeling well

before resuming your regimen. If you are new to exercise, begin conservatively with a low-intensity walking program, or simply use the stairs instead of the lift. Walking and other weight-bearing exercises help to build muscle strength and bone density—an important consideration for people with IBD because the condition makes them susceptible to osteoporosis. Gentle stretch-and-tone exercise and exercising in warm water will provide relief for stiff and painful joints. The breathing techniques of yoga and tai chi are helpful for reducing stress. Most exercises are suitable for people with IBD, but you should consult your doctor before embarking on a program.

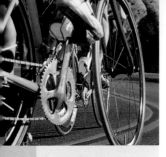

Bloating

BEST MOVES

walking

jogging

cycling

yoga

qigong

Pilates

Feeling bloated is the uncomfortable and sometimes painful sensation of having a stomach swollen by an excess of intestinal gas. Gas and abdominal cramps are usually symptomatic of digestive disorders caused by overeating, stress, or sensitivity to certain foods. Normally, food is digested and absorbed in the small intestine, but if sensitivity or intolerance interferes with this task, the unabsorbed food travels into the large intestine, where bacteria break it down and in the process release the gas that causes bloating.

Bloating is a common symptom of irritable bowel syndrome, because people with IBS are hypersensitive even to normal amounts of gas production. The bloated feeling experienced by many women around the time of their periods is caused by the increased fluid retention that arises from fluctuating hormone levels. Occasional bloating is normal and is usually dispelled within a few hours without treatment, but if you have persistent, unexplained bloating for more than four days, consult your doctor.

Why exercise helps

The old Chinese adage "100 steps after a meal" succinctly states the connection between physical activity and healthy digestion. A short walk after eating has a positive effect on the digestive system. Light exercise stimulates the secretion of the enzymes and hydrochloric acid needed to break down and absorb the food that has been ingested. A mild rhythmic movement, such as walking, also prompts the muscular contractions needed for bowel movements and for breaking down any large gas bubbles in the intestines. Avoid strenuous exercise, however, unless two hours have passed after eating a large meal. Otherwise blood will be diverted from the digestive tract, where it is needed to assist the speedy movement of food waste.

Yoga offers a number of simple poses designed to massage the digestive tract and relieve bloating (see pages 148–150). Qigong has a similarly benign effect on internal organs and stimulates blood circulation to promote healthy digestion. Both yoga and qigong calm the mind and reduce stress. Many digestive complaints are linked to emotional issues, especially anxiety and fear, which result in stomach pains and difficulty in eating.

Physical exercise alleviates the discomfort of menstrual bloating caused by fluid retention. Maintaining an exercise routine to encourage gastrointestinal health becomes even more important as we age and natural levels of hydrochloric acid and digestive enzymes decrease. Exercise helps to expand blood vessels and transport fluid more efficiently to the kidneys, from where it is excreted.

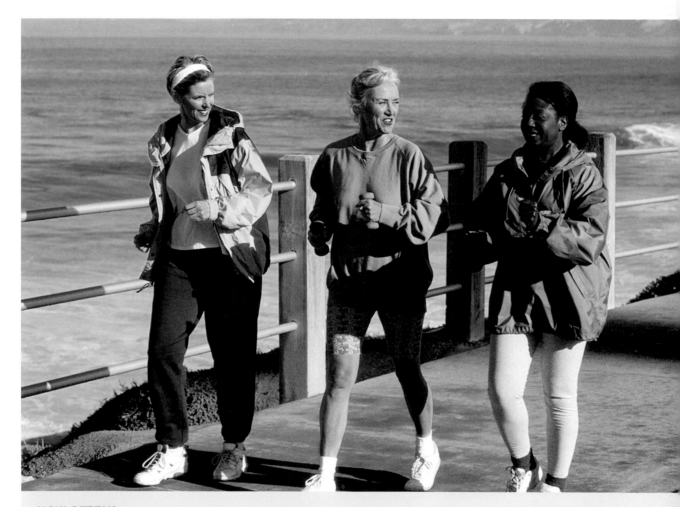

HOW OFTEN?

- Walk for 20 minutes after eating. A 20–30 minute brisk walk 4 times per week can improve bowel function.
- Practice qigong for 20 minutes every day for overall digestive health.
- As a preventive measure, exercise for a minimum of 30 minutes 5 days per week.
- Try to incorporate at least one session of yoga or Pilates into your weekly routine.
- A 30-minute workout or brisk walk 3 times per week will help to reduce fluid retention.

Walking is one of the best ways to help digestion and avoid bloating.

A sequence of yoga poses to relieve bloating

SIMPLE TWIST
Sit on a straight-backed, armless chair with both feet flat on the floor. Keeping your back straight and your pelvis level, twist your torso so your upper body is facing sideways. Help the twist by pulling on the back of the chair. Exhale during the twist. Then repeat on the other side.

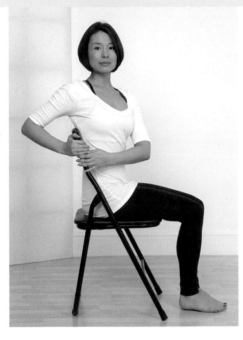

These poses massage the internal organs and endocrine glands, and improve digestion and elimination. Practice them in sequence 2 hours before or after eating—but don't do Shoulder Stand or Plow if you have high blood pressure.

WIND-RELIEVING POSE

Helps release trapped gas and stretches the lower back.

1. *Lie on your back. Inhale and bend your right leg up toward the chest. Interlace your fingers and hold the leg just below the kneecap.*

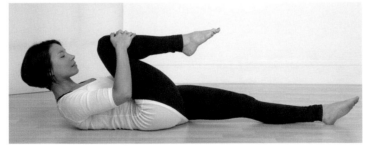

5. *Repeat on the other side. Alternate knees for 5 times or more, depending on the severity of symptoms.*

2. *Tuck your chin into your chest, raising your head slightly, and gently pull the knee in, hugging your thigh to your chest.*

3. *Breathe deeply, pressing your thigh against your chest as you inhale. Hold for 15 breaths.*

4. *Exhale and release arms and leg back to the floor.*

BELLY TWIST

Helps release trapped gas and stretches the lower back.

1. *Lie on your back and bring your arms out to the sides, with the palms facing down, in a T position. Bend both knees in toward the chest.*

2. *Exhale and drop both knees over to one side of your body, twisting the spine and lower back. Slide the knees as close to your arm as possible. Look at the opposite fingertips.*

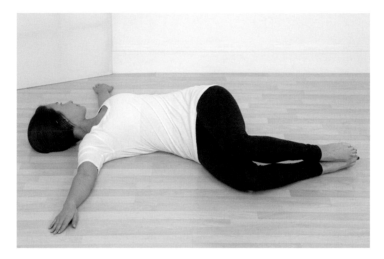

3. *Keep the shoulders flat to the floor, close your eyes, and relax into the posture. Let gravity pull the knees down.*

4. *Breathe and hold for 6–10 breaths.*

5. *Inhale and roll the hips back to the floor.*

6. *Repeat on the other side.*

SHOULDER STAND

1. *Lie on your back, arms alongside your body with palms down. Have a folded towel or mat under your neck for support. Bend the knees and kick and rock the legs up and back, bringing the bent knees to the forehead. Place hands under hips.*

2. *Bring your legs upright, straightening them above your head. Be sure to support the weight of your body with arms and shoulders. It is important not to put any weight on your neck.*

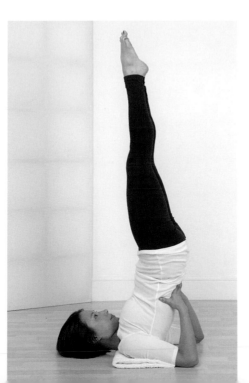

3. *Breathe and hold for up to 10 breaths.*

4. *To release, bend the knees back to the head, and carefully and slowly roll the spine back to the floor. Alternatively, before this, lower the legs over your head until your toes touch the floor in the Plow pose (see page 150).*

149

A sequence of yoga poses to relieve bloating continued

PLOW

Practicing this posture helps regulate the functioning of the kidneys, liver, and pancreas, and activates digestion. Do not do this pose if you have sciatica, backache, or high blood pressure.

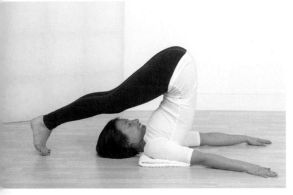

1. *Lie flat on your back, arms straight at your sides with the palms down. Bend the knees, bend the trunk upward, and kick and rock the legs up. As the legs pass the vertical position, curl the trunk so that the legs come down over your head and your toes touch the floor.*

2. *Keeping the legs straight, bend your arms and support your back with your hands.*

3. *Breathe and hold for up to 10 breaths.*

4. *Bend the knees back to the head, and carefully and slowly roll back down to the floor.*

Try something different
A simple qigong exercise to improve digestion

1. Stand comfortably with your feet shoulder width apart with palms placed lightly in front of your lower abdomen.

2. Direct your attention to your palms. Imagine a warm, golden light ("qi," or life force) radiating from them.

3. Inhale smoothly, without straining, and circle your palms up the left side of your abdomen. As you exhale, circle the palms down the right side of the abdomen. Make this circling motion—inhale up on the left, exhale down on the right—20 or 30 times. Picture golden rays of energy flowing from your palms into your abdomen. The golden energy, or qi, fills your internal organs, melting away obstructions and tension.

6. Change direction. Repeat, inhaling as your palms move up the right side of your abdomen and exhaling as they move down the left. Circle 20 or 30 times and imagine the qi radiating through your whole body, dissolving blockages and disease.

7. Let the qi radiate from your body and surround you, as if you were standing in a golden cocoon.

8. Bring your palms to rest again in front of your lower abdomen and imagine that you are holding a ball of golden light. Stand quietly for a minute or two, then open your palms and release the ball of light into the universe.

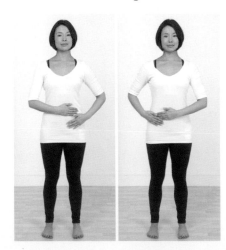

Chapter 8

Hormones

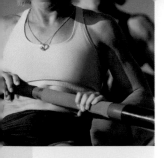

Diabetes

BEST MOVES

pump classes

circuit training

qigong

tai chi

walking

running

rowing

cycling

weight training

dancing

swimming

kickboxing

Pilates

high-intensity
interval training

Diabetes is characterized by a shortage of insulin, or a decreased ability to use insulin, which is a hormone that allows glucose (sugar) to enter cells and be converted to energy. When diabetes is not controlled, glucose and fats linger in the blood and eventually damage vital organs. There is no known way to prevent type 1 diabetes, which usually occurs in children and young adults, but type 2—which makes up the vast majority of diabetes cases—is strongly linked with lifestyle factors, such as lack of exercise and poor diet. Type 2 diabetes can cause high blood pressure, heart disease, kidney failure, and blindness.

A third form of diabetes, glucose intolerance, may arise during pregnancy. Gestational diabetes, as it is known, tends to affect women who are obese or have a family history of diabetes. Around half of those diagnosed with gestational diabetes will go on to develop type 2.

In 2009, Northwestern University researchers released the results of the longest observational study ever undertaken to investigate the relationship between cardiovascular fitness and the development of diabetes. They concluded that being aerobically fit was less important to the management of diabetes than losing weight. Sleep is also a significant factor. Too little sleep can have a hormonal impact on your nervous system that makes you more

sensitive to insulin. This greatly increases the risk of gaining excessive weight, as well as developing type 2 diabetes. People who sleep too much (nine or more hours) also have a higher risk of developing diabetes.

Why exercise helps

The onset of type 2 diabetes is fostered by a sedentary lifestyle and unhealthy eating habits. Regular exercise can have a dramatic and positive effect on the condition. It lowers blood sugar and lessens insulin resistance and the amount of fat in the liver. Physical activity improves muscle strength and aerobic capacity, and keeps in check the health complications that commonly lead people with type 2 diabetes to be at high risk of stroke and heart disease.

An exercise regimen that combines resistance training (lifting weights and leg-press exercises) with aerobic exercise is the most effective way to achieve the weight loss and muscle gain needed to control blood sugar. Some research suggests that even moderate amounts of exercise, such as walking, tai chi, and qigong, will start reducing the inflammation in visceral (stomach) fat that is linked with metabolic syndrome, a cluster of risk factors for heart disease and type 2 diabetes. A study conducted in Taiwan found that diabetes patients who performed tai chi for a few hours

HORMONES

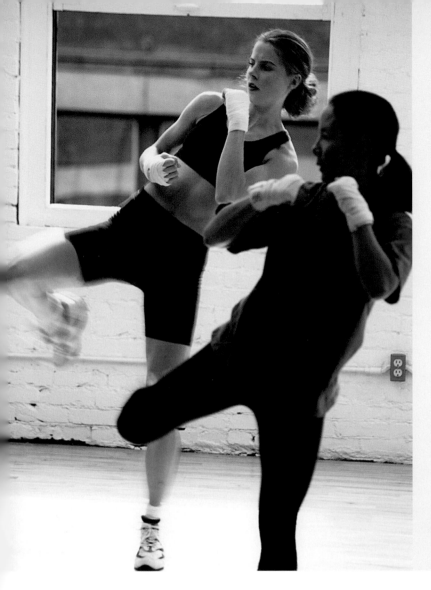

HOW OFTEN?

- Three hours per week of weight training combined with aerobic activity, such as kickboxing, burns body fat and can reduce the risk of type 2 diabetes by 58 percent. Gym circuit training and pump—a gym class that mixes weight training and aerobics—is ideal. Start with light weights.
- If you are new to exercise, walking is a good way to begin. Walking for 30–45 minutes on 5 days per week will reduce the likelihood of developing type 2 diabetes and heart disease.
- Go to a qigong or tai chi class at least once per week.
- Swimming and running are excellent for weight loss and muscle tone. To speed up fat loss, try high-intensity interval training once or twice per week, if your health status allows it (see page 154).

each week over a three-month period showed significant improvements in their health. The researchers concluded that tai chi encourages blood glucose levels to fall and improves blood glucose metabolism, which boosts the body's immune response.

People with type 1 diabetes must manage exercise differently. Exercise can actually raise blood sugar levels if it is started when the blood sugar level is 300 or higher. Those with insulin-dependent type 1 diabetes should test their blood sugar around 30 minutes before exercising, and then five minutes before exercising, to determine if their blood glucose level will allow them to exercise at that time or whether they need a source of quick-acting carbohydrates to prevent their blood sugar from dipping too low during their exercise session.

Above: *Aerobic activities, such as kickboxing, control weight gain, which protects against the onset of type 2 diabetes.*

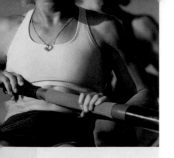

Diabetes continued

Regular exercise can have a dramatic and positive effect on diabetes. It lowers blood sugar and lessens insulin resistance and the amount of fat in the liver.

High-intensity interval training

Also known as HIIT, high-intensity interval training is a specialized form of workout that involves short intervals of maximum-intensity exercise separated by longer intervals of low- to moderate-intensity exercise—for example, cycling or running hard for three or four minutes, then recovering for two minutes with an interval of easy cycling or running. You need to put in your maximum effort during the high-intensity phase. Recovery periods should not last long enough for your pulse to return to its resting rate. This alternating fast-slow technique can dramatically improve cardiovascular fitness and raise the body's potential to burn fat.

A vigorous workout builds new lean muscle fiber, and the more muscle fiber you have, the more efficiently your body metabolizes carbohydrates and fat. If you are sedentary and overweight, those carbohydrates stagnate in your blood in the form of blood sugar and fat, which can cause metabolic syndrome, obesity, insulin resistance, high cholesterol, and elevated triglycerides—all markers for heart disease and diabetes.

A cautionary note

High-intensity interval training isn't for everyone, though. HIIT melts fat cells by pushing up your heart rate and you need to have a reasonable level of fitness before embarking on this kind of exercise. Anyone with heart disease or high blood pressure, or over the age of 60, should consult a doctor before starting interval training. For more about HIIT and weight control, see pages 156–160.

HOW OFTEN?
- If you are in good health, try high-intensity interval training for 20 minutes once per week and gradually build up to 3 times per week. HIIT is physically demanding, so be careful not to overdo it.
- Runners can alternate walking and sprints. Swimmers can complete a couple of fast laps, then 4 more slowly. Cyclists can do 2 sets of sprints followed by 2 sets of slow cycling. Don't do interval work on consecutive days.

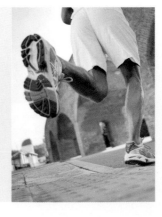

Why you need to shift abdominal fat

"Apple-shaped" people, who carry fat in the abdomen, have a higher risk of heart disease, diabetes, and other health problems than "pear-shaped" people, who tend to store fat in the hips and thighs. Although most people are more concerned about subcutaneous fat—the visible "spare tire" around the middle—the danger lies with visceral fat, which is located behind the abdominal wall and surrounds the internal organs.

Visceral fat cells in the abdomen secrete inflammatory molecules that enter the bloodstream and increase the risk of heart disease and diabetes. There is also evidence that inflammation plays a role in cancer and in aging.

The key to fighting molecular inflammation lies in increasing your metabolism—the rate at which your body burns fat. If you've got a fat stomach and you want to decrease your risk of getting diabetes, heart disease, and a raft of other disorders, you need to shrink your stomach's fat cells by elevating your metabolism. To do that you have to make a physical effort—combining resistance training with a cardio workout—that works muscle groups hard enough to raise the metabolism for several hours after exercising.

How to shift abdominal fat

- Resistance exercise is more beneficial than aerobic exercise for fat loss.
- Resistance training using weights, resistance bands, or exercise machines is the key to losing stomach fat. Lifting weights builds lean muscle mass, which burns calories and raises metabolism. The weights don't have to be heavy. Weight loss results come from the number of repetitions and sets that you do.
- There is no way to target specific areas of fat. Ab exercises alone will not shift fat from your mid-section. Do full-body circuit training 3 times per week, which combines resistance training and aerobics. Working legs, back, and chest will burn more calories and raise metabolism more than an isolated approach to training. Dancing and Pilates are also great all-body workouts.
- As the day passes, metabolic rate dips and calories aren't processed as efficiently. Some people find that exercising in the evening is more effective for burning calories because it reverses metabolic decline.
- To achieve faster results, try high-intensity interval training for 20 minutes on at least 3 days per week.
- Eat 4–6 small meals each day, with plenty of lean protein. Protein maintains muscle mass, which increases your metabolism and helps you burn fat faster.
- Accept that losing stomach fat may take some time, but your persistence will be rewarded.

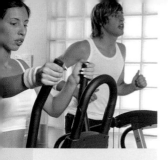

Weight control

BEST MOVES

resistance training

full-body circuit training

walking

running

stair climbing

hiking

cycling

swimming

aqua aerobics

rowing

step aerobics

elliptical trainer

golf

gardening

dancing

football

racket sports

tai chi

yoga

high-intensity interval training

HORMONES

People build up excessive fat in their bodies when the foods they consume convert to more energy than they expend. The result is weight gain that is harmful to health and has an adverse effect on life expectancy.

Degrees of being overweight are usually measured by Body Mass Index (BMI), which takes into account a person's weight, height, and gender. A body weight 20 percent higher than normal is an indication of obesity. Unhealthy diets and lack of physical exercise are key factors in the increase of obesity and other metabolic disorders in modern societies.

People who have become obese, or excessively overweight, have high levels of inflammatory molecules, which are secreted by fat tissue, circulating in their blood. This inflammation triggers the systemic diseases linked with metabolic syndrome, such as type 2 diabetes and heart disease.

Lack of sleep, along with a junk diet and a sedentary lifestyle, can also contribute to weight gain. If you don't get enough sleep, your body loses the ability to regulate its appetite. Sleep deprivation lowers your levels of leptin, the hormone that tells your body when it has had enough to eat, and increases levels of another hormone, ghrelin, which stimulates appetite. Not only does lack of sleep trigger hormonal imbalances

that encourage weight gain, but it leaves you feeling too tired to exercise. Sleep right, eat right, and exercise. That's the only way to burn fat.

Why exercise helps

Moderate intensity: Even moderate amounts of exercise can reduce fat, check insulin sensitivity, and improve heart health. A study by the University of Illinois found that moderate exercise helps to decrease, or prevent, the risk of developing life-threatening diseases, even when obesity is still present. That is, even though you may be overweight, just getting started on an exercise program is doing you good.

When it comes to achieving long-term weight loss, there is still debate about whether moderate or high-intensity exercise is the most effective. Advocates of moderate exercise say that to burn calories, muscle movements don't have to be extreme. Leisure and domestic activities, such as gardening, golf, hiking, housework, and polishing the car, do the same job of controlling weight as sweaty gym sessions. What really makes a difference is reining in your eating.

High intensity: Advocates of high-intensity exercise say that harder workouts really do accelerate improvements in body composition. Light exercise will keep burning calories

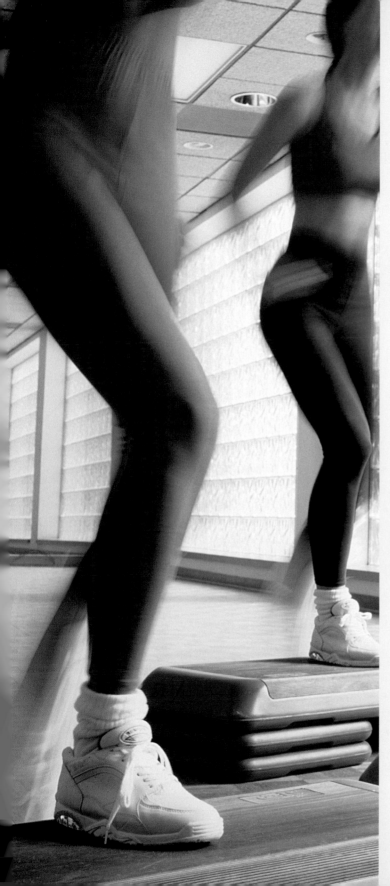

HOW OFTEN?

- To maintain a healthy weight, the American Nutrition and Health Foundation recommends the average adult performs 30 minutes of moderate aerobic activity on 5 days per week; or 20 minutes of vigorous aerobic activity on 3 days per week; or 30 minutes of moderate exercise on 2 days per week plus 20 minutes of aerobic activity on another 2 days per week.
- Overweight and obese persons may need up to 5 hours of exercise per week to lose weight.
- Depending on your level of fitness, begin with 5 minutes of walking daily and work up to 60 minutes, until you are fit enough to alternate walking with 60-minute sessions of other aerobic exercise and resistance training.

Note that moderate aerobic activity means exercise that elevates the heart rate enough to make you feel warm. Examples are brisk walking, yoga, recreational swimming, carrying children, and climbing stairs. Vigorous aerobic activity increases heart rate enough to cause rapid breathing and sweating. Examples are running, swimming laps, cycling fast, and running up stairs.

Left: *Performing step aerobics for 20 minutes three times per week helps the body maintain a healthy weight.*

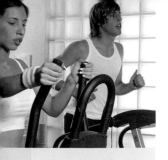

The best kind of fat attack of all is resistance training combined with high intensity interval training. This approach rapidly elevates metabolism and is a fierce burner of calories.

Weight control continued

for a few minutes post-workout, but vigorous exercise keeps burning calories for several hours afterward.

The term "high intensity" is relative to your capacity for exercise. In the case of a very overweight person, high intensity may mean walk-jogging, working out on a gym exercise machine, or, better yet, aqua aerobics. Aqua aerobics is a great way for overweight people to exercise. The buoyancy of the water alleviates stress on joints and makes the workout more comfortable. This can be a useful motivating factor to stick with an exercise routine.

Resistance training: A third school of thought maintains that you cannot successfully lose fat unless you do resistance/weight training. Resistance training increases muscle strength and endurance by using weights, weight machines, or resistance bands, although any activity involving effort that requires resistance, such as squats, push-ups, or lifting children, is included in the term resistance training.

Why is this technique so effective for weight loss? Because it builds muscle and muscle consumes calories. The more lean muscle you have, the more fat you will burn during activity. A resistance workout also raises your metabolism for a prolonged period of time, which lets you go on burning calories hours after the workout. If you circuit trained hard

in the gym for an hour at seven in the morning, you would still be burning calories when the afternoon rolled around. The harder you work, the longer this supercharge lasts. Aerobic workouts don't have the same after-burn as a resistance workout.

Be aware that you probably won't weigh less through resistance training, because you are gaining muscle. Judge your weight loss results by the fact that your clothes are looser, your measurements are less, and your body definition is more toned and shapely.

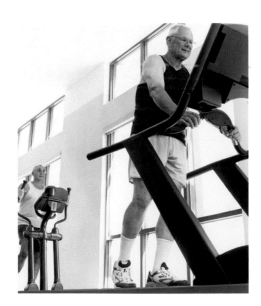

Walking or jogging on the gym treadmill is good for those with weight to lose who prefer the discipline of a gym routine to devising a route outdoors.

Pressed for time?

If you are overweight with very little time to spare, the most efficient way you can shift fat is to do one hour of metabolic resistance training three times per week in a gym. You can break that down into six sessions of 30 minutes each, or four of 45 minutes, or whatever combination works for you. Just make sure it adds up to three hours. Five hours of weight training won't make you lose more weight than three hours, so just do three hours. This type of exercise involves such activities as circuit training, supersets (working on the same group of muscles by repeating the same exercises in rapid succession), and barbell complexes. For these, use the bar with no weights on the ends to start with. Barbell complexes consist of up to 10 exercises, such as dead lifts, squats, and presses, in sets of six repetitions. You move from one exercise to the next without ever taking a break or letting go of the bar.

If you can carve out a little more time to up the rate at which you are losing weight, try adding one or two sessions of aerobic exercise per week.

High-intensity interval training?

One way of achieving more dramatic weight loss and fitness results is to add two 20-minute sessions of aerobic high-intensity interval training (HIIT) to

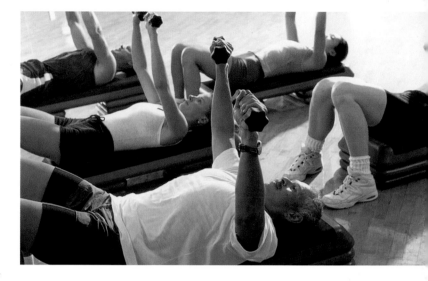

your three hours of resistance training. HIIT is a tough workout, alternating short intervals of maximum effort with slightly longer intervals of moderate work (for more about HIIT see page 154). The high-intensity phase should be long and strenuous enough to make you out of breath, usually about one to four minutes of exercise, but you can do shorter, more frequent bursts of maximum-intensity activity, such as sprinting for 20 seconds and jogging/walking for 60 seconds, and repeating that 15 to 20 times per session. HIIT increases the amount of calories you burn during your exercise session and afterward because it increases the length of time it takes your body to recover from each exercise session. To benefit from HIIT, you need

A program of weight training adding up to three hours per week will help shift unwanted pounds. Add some aerobic activity to make faster progress.

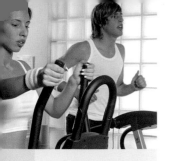

The best kind of fat attack of all is resistance training combined with high intensity interval training. This approach rapidly elevates metabolism and is a fierce burner of calories.

Weight control continued

to push yourself past the upper end of your aerobic zone and allow your body to replenish your anaerobic energy system during the recovery intervals. In other words, you need to work at your physical maximum during the intense phase. That is why HIIT is not for beginner exercisers or people with health risks. If you have high blood pressure, heart problems, or other health issues that could compromise your ability to do very intense exercise, or if you are not very fit, don't attempt HIIT. In any case, don't begin a HIIT program for weight loss unless you can already exercise at

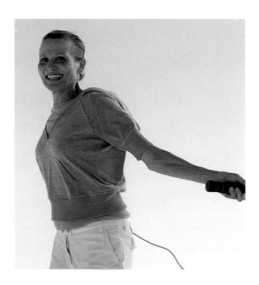

Jumping rope raises the body's metabolic rate, and burns calories, helping you manage your weight.

70 percent of your maximum heart rate without feeling wiped out. If you want to get involved in HIIT, having first checked with your doctor, you should consult with a trainer at your gym to devise an interval program that works for you and allows you to build up your HIIT training gradually over several weeks.

Eating and exercising

If you work out physically, you're going to get hungry and eat more. That's what happens. But you don't want to undermine the good work you've done in the gym by chowing down on a cheeseburger and fries. People who start running are often surprised to find that they haven't lost any weight—at least, in the first few weeks. In fact, a lot of people gain weight. That is because new runners often have a greater appetite than before they started running and they simply eat more of everything. Just because you are exercising doesn't mean that you can eat food crammed with calories and still expect to lose weight. Even if you aren't doing high-intensity exercise, eating a pre-workout snack and then eating a small, healthy meal immediately after a workout can keep you from overeating later in the day.

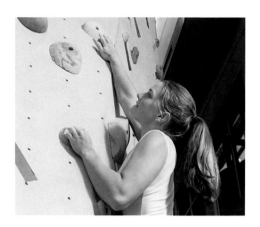

During an hour of rock climbing, a person weighing 154 pounds (70 kg) will burn an average of 775 calories.

Walking

People who are significantly overweight will find that walking is a benign way to embark on a weight-loss exercise program.

- Begin by walking as briskly as you can for five to 10 minutes. Take a rest of a few minutes and then walk for a further five minutes. Walk every other day, alternating walking with brief rest periods. Add gradual increments of 30 seconds to your walking. As the duration of your walk lengthens, try to walk a little more briskly as well. At the end of your walk do some stretching to relax your muscles.
- For the first eight weeks of your walking program, don't walk on consecutive days. Assuming that you

Try something different

INDOOR ROCK CLIMBING FOR A TOTAL-BODY WORKOUT

Indoor rock climbing is an exciting activity that involves climbing up a wall in a controlled environment that simulates the experience of outdoor rock climbing. The wall is usually around 30 feet (9 meters) high and has a variety of resin hand and footholds. Climbers wear a safety harness to protect them from injury if they fall. You can find indoor climbing walls at climbing centers and at some gyms and fitness centers.

As a beginner, you will first be given a skills and safety lesson by a qualified instructor and then you can get started. The benefits of regular climbing are tremendous. Indoor climbing is not only fun, especially as a joint activity to be shared with family and friends, but it is a calorie-consuming, total-body workout that helps you to lose weight.

Climbing develops coordination, endurance, strength, flexibility, and balance. As an added bonus, indoor climbing is mentally stimulating, because you have to figure out the best climbing route to the top of the wall. You get a great feeling of accomplishment when you reach the top—and that will motivate you to do more and maintain your fitness.

are making a real effort with each walking session, your body needs recovery time. After two or three weeks, by which time your body will be used to exercising, try some gentle alternative activity on your non-walking days, such as aqua aerobics, tai chi, or yoga. Make sure you have a day off from exercise once a week.

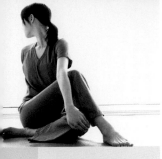

Thyroid imbalance

BEST MOVES

yoga

walking

resistance training

cycling

dancing

rowing

swimming

Pilates

Many weight-related problems can be improved by boosting the function of the thyroid gland. This butterfly-shaped gland in the throat regulates energy levels, body temperature, and weight, and has been linked to mood and depression.

Low thyroid activity (hypothyroidism) causes fatigue, weight gain, hair loss, dry skin, and constipation. People with hypothyroidism often feel tired or cold and have trouble sleeping. High thyroid activity (hyperthyroidism) causes weight loss, a racing heart, restlessness, frequent bowel movements, and tremors.

Medications, including synthetic hormones and radioactive iodine, are usually prescribed to treat thyroid imbalance, but physical activity is essential to deal with the weight problems that are associated with this condition.

Why exercise helps

Resistance training is ideal exercise for people with thyroid problems who are battling weight gain, because it helps to build calorie-burning lean muscle. Resistance training means any exercise that causes the muscles to contract against an external resistance, such as dumbbells and barbells, your own body weight, and various gym machines.

In yoga, the practice of certain postures has long been recommended in order to maintain a balanced thyroid function. For an underactive thyroid (hypothyroidism) try poses that place gentle pressure on the neck or throat and stimulate blood flow to the thyroid gland, such as Shoulder Stand (see page 166), Bridge (see page 72), and Plow (see page 150). People with an overactive thyroid (hyperthyroidism) tend to have a rapid or irregular heart rate. They may benefit from calming, restorative yoga poses, such as Reclining Cobbler (see page 66), Legs Up The Wall (see page 73), Supported Corpse, and Supported Child's Pose.

Yoga adepts also believe that an under- or overactive thyroid occurs because of deficient energy in the throat chakra. In Eastern philosophy, a chakra is an energy center in the body associated with particular physical functions and with specific life issues. Shoulder openers and poses that stretch the neck, such as Camel (see page 72), Bridge, Shoulder Stand, and Plow, are considered to help a deficient throat chakra.

Opposite: *The practice of yoga is believed to promote good thyroid function. Poses such as Shoulder Stand (see also page 166) stimulate the thyroid gland.*

HORMONES

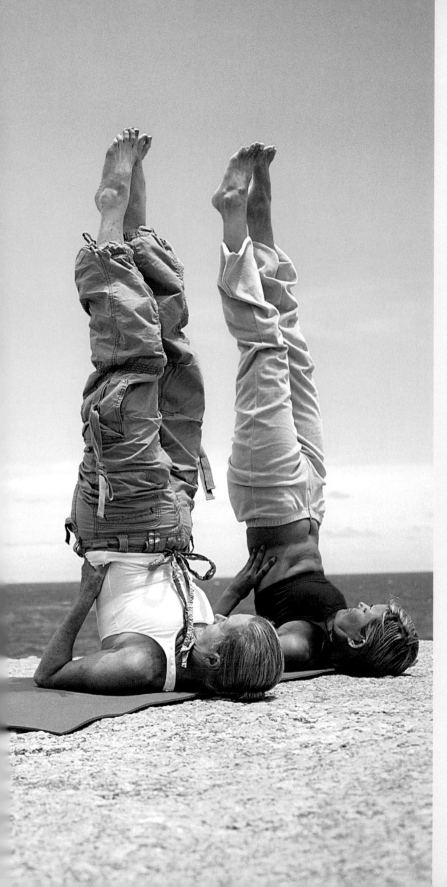

HOW OFTEN?

- Aim to maintain an exercise program of 30–60 minutes per day for 4 or 5 days per week to correct imbalances in your insulin and leptin levels. (Leptin is a hormone that helps to regulate body weight by controlling appetite.)
- Practice yoga at home for 30 minutes on 3 days per week, or at a 1-hour class once a week.
- Walk for 30 minutes, alternating with a session of resistance training.
- For resistance training at home, do one set (8–12 repetitions) of 8–10 exercises for the major muscle groups on 2–3 days per week.

Note that some appropriate resistance-training exercises using free weights are: two-arm bent-over rows; upright rows; dumbbell or bar press; flyes; triceps press; kickbacks. You can use your own body weight to do push-ups, sit-ups, chin-ups, squat thrusts, lunges, and step-ups. The advantage of these exercises is that you can do most of them anywhere.

Circuit work to stimulate metabolism

People with sluggish thyroids often find it tough to lose weight. Circuit training is one of the most effective ways to elevate a slow metabolism because it combines the benefits of aerobic and strength exercises. If you don't have access to a gym or gym machines, you can get the same circuit-work benefit while you're out running in the park, or on a treadmill or stationary bike at home. Just do 2 minutes of aerobic exercise and then 2 minutes of weight-bearing exercises, such as leg raises, lunges, and push-ups, which work the main muscle groups. Lunges strengthen and firm legs and buttocks. Push-ups strengthen and tone upper arms, shoulders, and back. Leg raises strengthen abdominals and the lower back.

TO DO A CIRCUIT:

- Walk or jog for 1–2 minutes.
- Stop and do 1–2 minutes of lunges, alternating legs.
- Walk or jog for another 2 minutes.
- Stop and do push-ups for 2 minutes.
- Walk or jog for 2 minutes.
- Stop and do 2 minutes of leg raises.
- Rest for 2 minutes.
- Repeat the circuit twice more.

As you become stronger, you can increase the duration of the strength-training intervals by adding more repetitions to the lunges, push-ups, and leg raises.

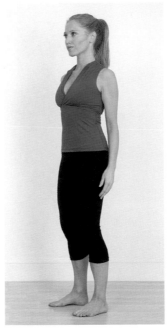

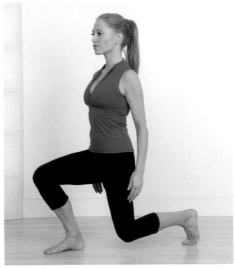

LEG LUNGES

1. *Do these leg lunges for 1–2 minutes on alternating legs. Begin by standing with your feet shoulder-width apart, with your hands at your sides. Inhale and step the left foot back.*

2. *Your left knee should be a little above the floor. Check that your right knee does not extend beyond the toes of your right foot. Keep your hands at your sides and look straight ahead.*

3. *Return the left leg to the starting position. Repeat with the right leg, and repeat, alternating right and left legs for 1–2 minutes.*

PUSH-UPS

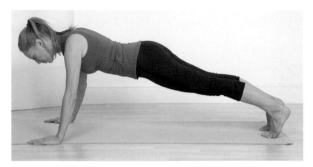

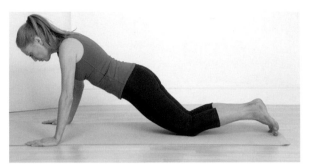

1. Lie face down and place your hands on the floor, parallel with your shoulders, palms down. Push up, lifting your legs and trunk off the floor. Keep your back and legs straight and toes curled under.

2. If a straight-arm push-up is too difficult, you can push up from your knees. Once you can do 20–25 knee push-ups on the floor, you are probably ready to do conventional push-ups.

LEG RAISES

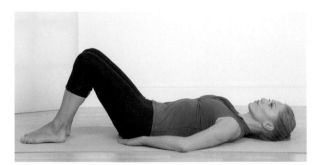

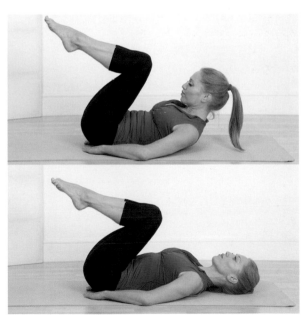

1. Lie on your back on a towel or mat. Place your hands under your buttocks, palms facing the floor, to protect your lower back.

2. Inhale and as you exhale bend your knees and raise them toward your chest while simultaneously lifting your head off the floor and tucking your chin into your chest.

3. Lower your head to the floor and straighten your legs, but do not let them touch the floor. Repeat as many times as possible for 1–2 minutes.

Yoga poses for thyroid imbalance

SHOULDER STAND

Fold two thick blankets into a square. Place the blankets at the back end of your mat. Lie down with your shoulders on the blankets, but your head off them. Bring your arms down alongside your body, keeping them close to your body. Keeping your legs together, swing your legs and hips up so your hips are stacked above your shoulders. Place your palms squarely on your lower back with fingers pointing up toward your heels. Tuck in your chin and nestle it right in the notch between your collarbones. Tuck your elbows in closely, making sure they are square to the sides of your body, not angling out. Hold this position for 23 breaths or more.

To come out of the position, bend your knees toward your forehead, hinging from your hips, using your abdominal muscles to roll your back and hips toward the floor. Once your hips are on the floor, straighten your legs out one at a time.

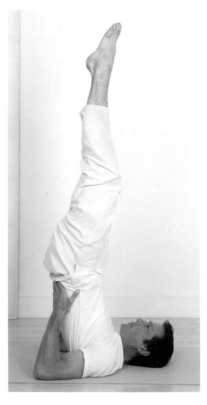

Shoulder Stand is considered to be the yoga pose of greatest benefit to the thyroid.

RECLINING COBBLER

This restorative posture helps regulate hormone production. Take a bolster and a folded blanket. Place the bolster behind you lengthwise and put the folded blanket on top of the bolster. Bring the soles of your feet together close to the groin, knees open to the sides (see top image). Lie back, with your spine supported on the bolster; rest your head on the blanket with your chin tucked in slightly. Relax your arms alongside your body, palms facing up, or resting on your abdomen. If your legs don't feel comfortable, cross your feet at the ankles (see lower image). Close your eyes, breathe calmly, and remain in this position for up to 15 minutes.

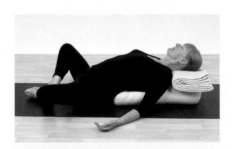

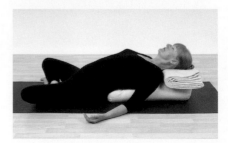

Chapter 9

Kidney, Liver, and Urinary

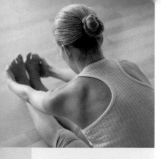

Stress incontinence

BEST MOVES

pelvic-floor exercises

Pilates

yoga "root lock"

Stress is the most common cause of urinary incontinence. The bladder leaks urine in response to sudden pressure from a physical activity, such as high-impact exercise, coughing, sneezing, sex, or laughing. It happens due to weakness in the pelvic floor—the "hammock" of muscles, ligaments, and tissues that supports the organs of the pelvis (the uterus, bladder, and rectum). It's the job of the pelvic floor to contract in order to close the bladder and the urethra (the tube that carries urine). Women are particularly susceptible to weak pelvic-floor muscles and stress incontinence, usually due to childbirth, aging, constipation, or being overweight.

Why exercise helps

Stress incontinence can be treated by practicing exercises designed to strengthen the muscles in the pelvic floor (see page 170). These are sometimes known as Kegel exercises, named after the doctor who devised them for women as a method of controlling incontinence following childbirth. If you get into a routine of doing pelvic-floor exercises during pregnancy and after giving birth, stress incontinence is less likely to develop later in life.

Regular Pilates is also effective for preventing or reversing stress incontinence, because Pilates exercises work to strengthen core muscles in the abdomen, including the pelvic floor.

Yoga uses a special technique called mula bandha, or root lock (the word "bandha" means to tighten) to contract the pelvic-floor muscles in order to build core strength, increase vitality, and enable the body to use less energy to hold a yoga posture. Engaging mula bandha is similar to doing Kegel exercises and effectively strengthens pelvic-floor muscles (see page 171). Ashtanga yoga employs mula bandha as a key factor in its practice.

If incontinence is a problem for you, you might want to exchange running or other high-impact aerobic exercise for one that is more bladder-friendly, such as swimming or cycling.

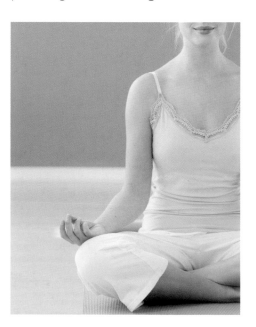

Yoga uses a "locking" technique to contract the pelvic-floor muscles.

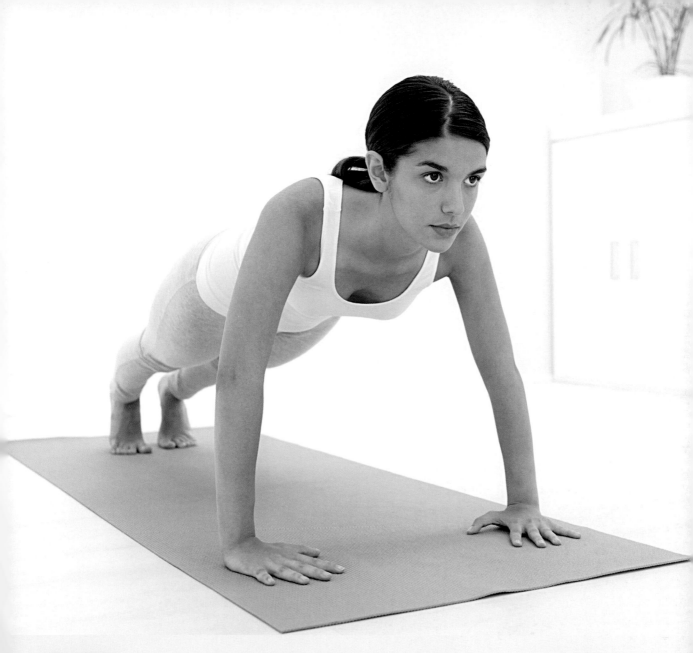

HOW OFTEN?

■ Pelvic-floor exercises need to be done regularly for 5 minutes at least 3 times per day. It takes 6–20 weeks for most women with stress incontinence to notice a change in urine loss. Once incontinence stops, continue to do one or two 5-minute bouts of pelvic-floor exercise each day to keep the muscles toned and prevent incontinence from returning.

Exercises that promote core stability can help prevent stress incontinence—the Plank helps build strong abdominals (see page 128.)

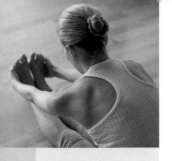

Women are particularly susceptible to weak pelvic-floor muscles and stress incontinence, usually as a result of childbirth, aging, constipation, or being overweight.

Stress incontinence continued

How to do pelvic-floor exercises

It is important to exercise the correct muscles. The sensation of exercising your pelvic floor is an internal one—it does not involve squeezing muscles in your buttocks, thighs, or stomach.

Finding the muscles

- Sit on a chair with your knees slightly apart. Imagine you are trying to stop passing gas. You will have to tighten the muscle just above the entrance to the anus. You should feel some movement in the muscle. Don't clench your buttocks or tense your thighs or stomach. Breathe slowly and deeply.
- Now imagine you are passing urine and need to stop the flow. You will find yourself using the pelvic-floor muscles nearer to the vagina. To check that you have found the right muscle to exercise, lie down and put your finger in your vagina and squeeze as if you are trying to stop urine from coming out. If you feel a little muscular pressure around your finger, you've found the right muscles.

Doing the exercises

- Sit, stand, or lie with your knees slightly apart. Slowly tighten your pelvic-floor muscles as firmly as you can. Hold for five seconds, breathing deeply and slowly. Relax. Repeat at least five times. These are called slow pull-ups. As the muscles become stronger, increase the length of time you hold each slow pull-up up to 10 seconds.
- Tighten your pelvic-floor muscles again and release immediately. Repeat at least five times. These are called fast pull-ups.
- Alternate five slow pull-ups and five fast pull-ups for five minutes.
- To achieve the desired result, pelvic-floor exercises need to be done three times a day. Aim to do each five-minute bout of exercise in a different position—sitting, standing, or lying down.
- In addition to scheduled practice time, try to get into the habit of doing the exercises at any time—for instance, when sitting in your car waiting for a light to change, or while talking on the phone.

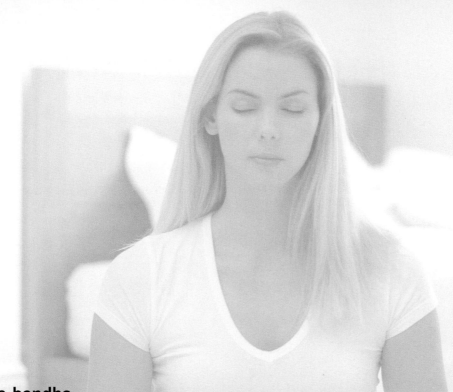

Mula bandha

The practice of mula bandha tones the urogenital organs, strengthens sphincter muscles, and stimulates intestinal contractions. But there is an added dimension to engaging mula bandha since, according to yogic philosophy, bandhas subtly influence the chakras to open and thus encourage energy flow.

- Sit in a relaxed posture on the floor with legs crossed if you are able. Otherwise sit on a chair. Rest the palms of your hands on your knees and close your eyes.
- Inhale deeply. As you exhale, gently contract the muscles around your anus. Keep breathing calmly.
- Direct your attention toward the pubic bone. Concentrate on the sensation of pulling up the perineum (the area between the anus and genitals) toward the abdomen, as if you were trying to stop urinating. The sensation should be one of gentle squeezing and lifting. Your effort should not be so great that it interferes with your breathing.
- As you pull up the pelvic floor, you should feel a little tightening (but not tensing) in the lower deep abdominal muscles. Hold the contraction for up to 10 seconds without holding your breath. Breathe easy.
- Release the contraction and repeat up to 10 times.
- When you find it easy to "switch on" mula bandha, you can engage it while you are doing yoga poses. It's a brilliant maintenance plan for your pelvic floor.

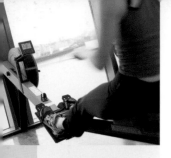

Urinary tract infections

BEST MOVES

pelvic-floor exercises

Pilates

walking

rowing

cycling

resistance training

qigong

tai chi

yoga

Symptoms of urinary tract infections (UTI) affect both men and women, but women are 10 times more likely to contract one of these infections. That is because a woman's urethra (the tube along which urine travels) is shorter than a man's, and it allows bacteria to reach the bladder more easily. Also, the closeness of a woman's urethra to her rectum can encourage cross-infection, and bacteria that are normally found in the gastrointestinal tract are the cause of most UTIs.

Symptoms include a pressing need to urinate more often than usual, an urge to urinate but not being able to, and a burning sensation when you do urinate. If an infection in the urethra is not treated—it requires a visit to the doctor and, usually, a course of antibiotics—it may develop into a bladder infection (cystitis) or a serious kidney infection (pyelonephritis), accompanied by fever, shivering, vomiting, and pain in the lower back or abdominal area.

Why exercise helps

Mobility helps your bladder to function efficiently, so even though the symptoms of a UTI cause discomfort, you will benefit from exercise. Exercise will also help relieve the stress of having a UTI. Keeping pelvic-floor muscles toned by doing regular pelvic-floor exercises (see pages 168–171) decreases the risk of contracting a UTI. Perform pelvic-floor exercises on an empty bladder. Pilates is an excellent activity for maintaining a toned pelvic floor and lower back, which helps keep the urogenitary area in good condition.

HOW OFTEN?
- Exercise for at least 30 minutes 3–5 times per week to maintain a degree of fitness that helps support the immune system and keep infections at bay.
- Take at least one Pilates or yoga class per week for core strength and a strong lower back.
- Do pelvic-floor exercises (see page 170) at least once daily.

Opposite: *Even regular dog-walking helps maintain basic fitness levels, boosting the immune system against potential infections.*

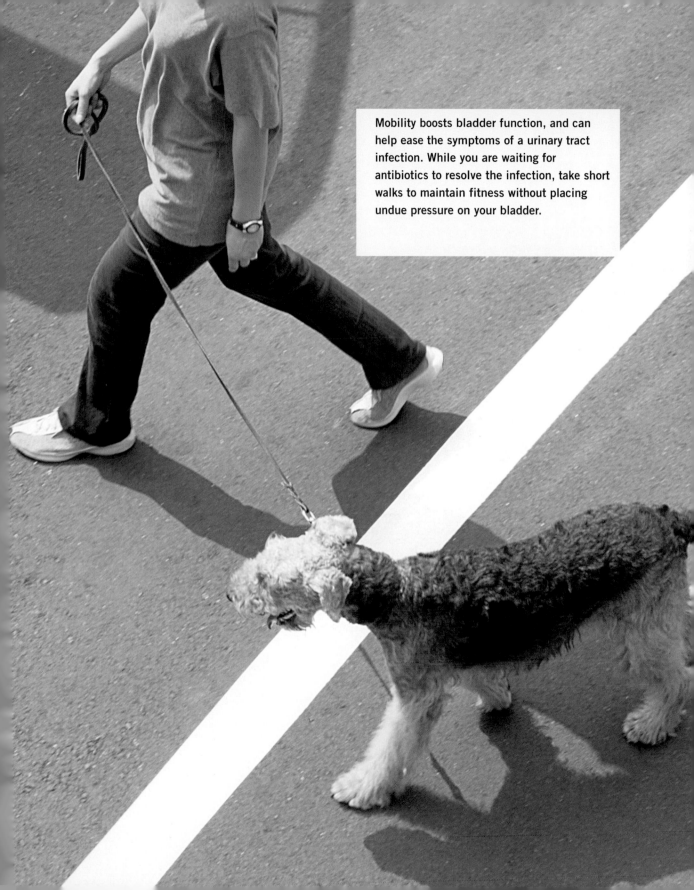

Mobility boosts bladder function, and can help ease the symptoms of a urinary tract infection. While you are waiting for antibiotics to resolve the infection, take short walks to maintain fitness without placing undue pressure on your bladder.

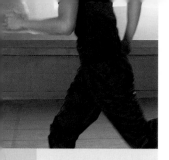

BEST MOVES

qigong

yoga

tai chi

resistance
training

walking

cycling

running

dancing

jumping on a
rebounder

Liver congestion

The liver performs many vital functions including cleansing the blood of toxins and regulating hormones. Its efficiency affects emotional states and mental activities. When stress, poor diet, or excessive use of alcohol or drugs damage the liver, its ability to cleanse the blood is diminished. Blood circulation becomes sluggish and the capacity to transport oxygen and nutrients is reduced, resulting in undernourished tissue and organ cells. Fatigue, depleted energy levels, low thyroid activity, and weight gain are all symptoms of a congested liver. According to traditional Chinese medicine, depression is an indication of blocked liver energy—and Chinese medicine and yogic philosophy both associate a damaged liver with the emotions of anger, resentment, and bitterness. Fortunately, the liver has strong regenerative powers and can be restored to optimal functioning.

Why exercise helps

Many people with a congested liver struggle with chronic tiredness, which may make the prospect of exercise seem

HOW OFTEN?

- **Up to 30 minutes of moderate exercise daily is ideal, at an intensity that promotes the deep breathing needed to enhance the circulatory system and detoxify the liver.**
- **Jump on a rebounder or Bosu Ball for 5–20 minutes per day.**
- **Daily qigong or tai chi.**
- **Three sessions of ashtanga, power, or Bikram yoga per week.**

Qigong helps stimulate the liver and boosts energy levels.

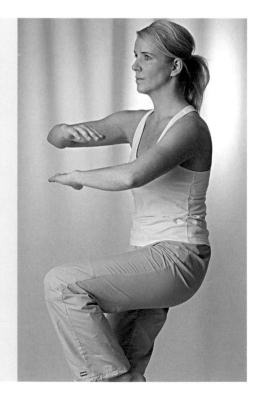

daunting. However, physical activity is the best way to combat the fatigue and feelings of sluggishness that accompany liver congestion. Exercise promotes liver health by moving the abdominal muscles and diaphragm. As the diaphragm expands the chest, it compresses the abdominal cavity. The gentle compression of the liver caused by each breath, and the pumping action of muscles, stimulates the circulation of blood and lymph through the liver.

"Bouncy," high-impact exercise, such as running and jumping, along with deep breathing, are especially useful for assisting the circulation of waste products through the liver. Swimming is also helpful, because it uses all the muscles and combines rhythmic breathing and movement.

According to traditional Chinese medicine, physical activity, such as qigong and tai chi, or any exercise that involves deep breathing and stretching, should be undertaken in the morning to get "stagnant" blood moving from the liver. Sweating toxins out through the skin also assists liver health. The skin's sweat glands excrete five to 10 percent of all metabolic wastes. Vigorous forms of yoga, such as ashtanga, power, and Bikram, all make use of sweating to cleanse the body of toxins.

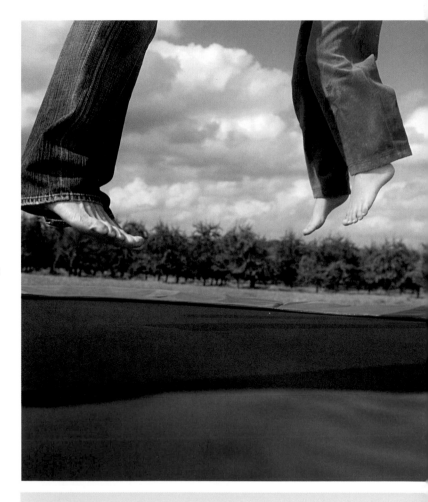

REBOUNDING

Jumping up and down on a rebounder, or mini trampoline, is considered the most efficient way of stimulating the lymphatic system to eliminate toxins. You can also jump on a Bosu Ball—half of a Swiss ball on a flat rubber platform. Its name is an acronym of Both Sides Up or Both Sides Utilized—you can do exercises on the flat platform and also on the soft, dome-shaped side. Gently bounce up and down on the rebounder, or the ball, working up to 20-minute sessions, daily if possible.

Exercises to help liver congestion

YOGIC FIRE BREATHING FOR LIVER PURIFICATION

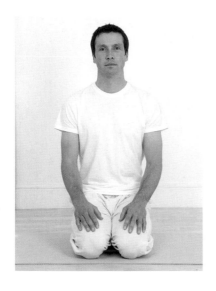

1. *Sit in Thunderbolt pose—with ankles and big toes together, touching the ground, sit on the heels.*

2. *Keeping the toes together, separate the knees as far as possible. Place both hands on the knees and lean the upper half of the body forward slightly, keeping the arms straight.*

3. *Open the mouth and extend the tongue. Breathe rapidly in and out by contracting and expanding the abdomen. You should sound like a dog panting. Repeat this rapid breathing 25 times.*

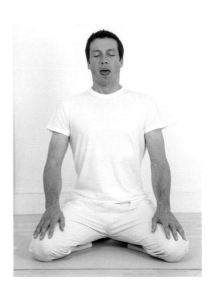

MERIDIAN STRETCH TO STIMULATE THE LIVER

1. *Sit on the floor with back straight and legs stretched straight out in front, toes pointing up.*

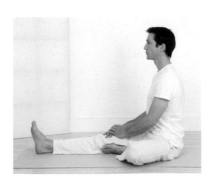

2. *Bend one leg and place the sole of the foot against the inner side of the opposite knee.*

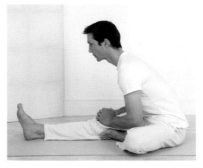

3. *Rest both hands on the knee of the straight leg. Keeping your back straight, begin to move your upper body forward and back in a slow, rocking motion.*

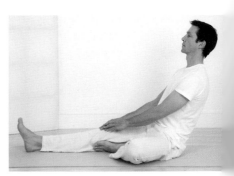

4. *Continue for at least a minute, breathing slowly and deeply. Repeat the exercise with the other leg.*

Chapter 10

Sleep

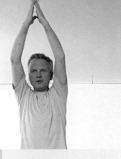

Insomnia

BEST MOVES

yoga

qigong

tai chi

moderate, aerobic activity

Insomnia is a sleep disorder in which a person has trouble falling asleep or staying asleep, and the sleep is of poor quality. About 30 percent of adults have insomnia. It is more common among older people and women, and people experiencing pain from medical conditions. Stress can cause a disturbed sleep pattern that lasts for several weeks or months, but chronic sleeplessness that does not resolve itself on its own can lead to short- and long-term health problems, such as anxiety disorders and depression. People who suffer from insomnia also have raised blood pressure at night, which, over time, can lead to heart problems.

Why exercise helps

Exercise improves sleep by producing a significant rise in body temperature, followed by a compensatory drop a few hours later. The drop in body temperature, which persists for two to four hours after exercise, makes it easier to fall asleep and stay asleep.

Regular aerobic exercise oxygenates the blood and reduces feelings of stress

Try something different

YOGA NIDRA

This is a state of conscious deep sleep and profound relaxation of mind and body. During the practice of yoga nidra, a person appears to be sleeping, but the consciousness is functioning at a deep level of awareness. The aim of the practice is to release muscular, mental, and emotional tensions. It is a powerful and effective way of accessing and altering stuck patterns of behavior that may be contributing to difficulties with sleeping.

Yoga Nidra is practiced in a dimly lit room. After some stretching to loosen up the body, you lie on a mat on the floor with your palms facing up. You choose a resolution or an intention—a behavioral or emotional tendency that you would like to alter—and repeat it mentally.

An instructor asks you to direct your attention to various parts of the body and relax them. As the body gradually relaxes, so does the mind, and space opens up mentally for new, fresh patterns to be laid down—such as learning to sleep.

As the instructor guides you through counting breaths, image visualizations, and other such practices, you repeat your resolution mentally. At the end of the session, your mind slowly returns to awareness of the present moment, feeling refreshed and recharged.

and anxiety, as well as helping to burn calories. Many people with chronic insomnia struggle with weight gain because sleep deprivation disrupts the production of hormones associated with feeling hungry and with metabolism. Activities that use leg muscles, such as jogging, swimming, cycling, dancing, riding a stationary bicycle, using a treadmill, and walking, are especially effective in combating sleeplessness.

A Brazilian study that looked at the effectiveness of using physical exercise to treat insomnia found that moderate exercise led to a significant increase in the total sleep time of participants, and reduced the length of time it took for them to fall asleep.

According to Chinese traditional medicine, chronic sleep disorders are caused by a yin-yang imbalance, arising from a weak liver, spleen, heart, or kidneys. The liver filters blood throughout the night, especially between one and three o'clock in the morning. Poor-quality sleep results when a weak or congested liver is struggling to function optimally. Attention to diet and regular practice of qigong or tai chi can correct the imbalance.

Meditation

People who can't sleep are in a 24-hour state of hyperarousal. Practicing deep-breathing relaxation techniques,

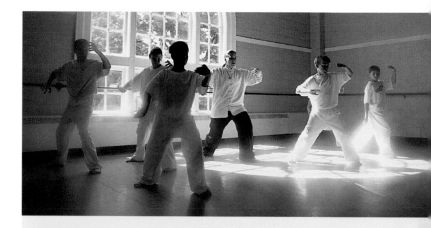

HOW OFTEN?

■ Engage in aerobic exercise on at least 4 days per week, for 20–30 minutes in the late afternoon, but not during the 4–6 hours before bedtime, and never just before you go to sleep. Exercise raises body temperature, and you sleep better when your body temperature is low. If you warm your body with a workout in the late afternoon, it will have cooled down by the time you are ready for sleep.

such as meditation, during the daytime can help lower mental overactivity and promote sleep at night.

A recent study at Northwestern Memorial Hospital in Illinois found that participants who practiced Kriya yoga for two months reported improved quality of sleep and mood. Kriya yoga, using hand gestures and simple movements, is a form of meditation that uses simple repetitive actions to internalize attention and reduce the "chattering" of the mind.

Above: *Moderate aerobic activity, such as qigong or tai chi, has a positive effect on insomnia. The key factors are that the exercise is regular and enjoyable.*

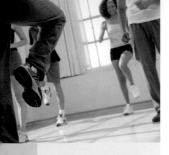

Sleep apnea

BEST MOVES

aerobic
exercise

mouth, throat,
and facial
exercises

Obstructive sleep apnea is a chronic disorder that can have serious consequences. Apnea means "no breath." People with this syndrome stop breathing for 10 to 30 seconds at a time while they are sleeping due to the complete or partial obstruction of the upper airway. This can happen if excess fat in the neck presses on the outside of the throat. The blockage stops the movement of air and the amount of oxygen in the blood drops. This causes the brain to send a signal to wake up and open the airway in the throat so that breathing can start again. Sometimes the body awakens with a gasp or a snort in order to resume breathing. The cycle may repeat itself as often as 50 or more times an hour. More rarely, sleep apnea may occur because the brain forgets to stimulate breathing.

Sleep apnea is defined by loud snoring, choking, or gasping during sleep, excessive daytime sleepiness, and other consequences of sleep disruption, such as lack of concentration, irritability, and changes in mood, including depression. It can be life threatening because it puts its sufferers at risk of stroke, heart failure, irregular heartbeat, high blood pressure, heartburn, and diabetes.

Why exercise helps

Exercises based on speech therapy can significantly reduce the severity of sleep apnea, snoring symptoms, daytime sleepiness, and sleep quality. These exercises—involving the tongue, soft palate, throat, and facial muscles (see pages 182–184)—remodel the muscles in the upper airway and help to decrease neck circumference. A recent study showed that snoring decreased and symptoms of obstructive sleep apnea improved when participants retrained their upper airway muscles by playing the didgeridoo—an Australian aboriginal wind instrument.

Since people with obstructive sleep apnea are usually carrying excess weight, especially around their necks, a weight-loss exercise program is frequently recommended as a basic treatment for the disorder. People who lose 10 percent of body weight can experience a 30 percent decrease in sleep apnea symptoms. A Sleep Heart Health study reported that vigorous physical activity for at least three hours each week helps to decrease disordered breathing during sleep.

Other studies have shown that even moderate exercise improves both subjective and objective measures of sleep. Recent data suggest that exercise can reduce the severity of

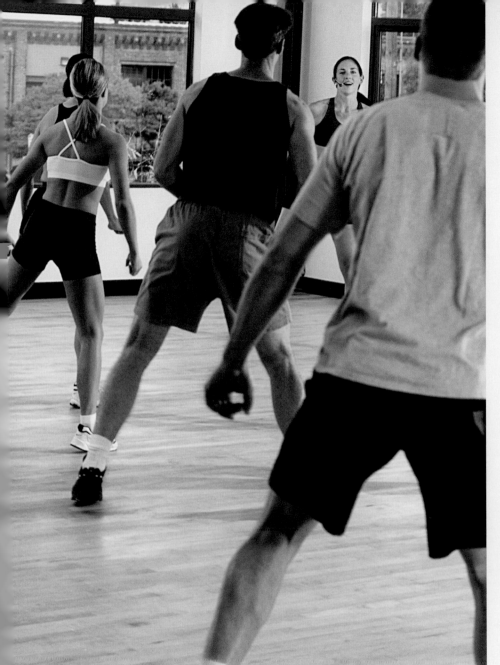

HOW OFTEN?

- Take aerobic exercise for 30 minutes per day on 5 days per week, at least 4–6 hours before bedtime and preferably in the late afternoon.
- Exercises involving the tongue, soft palate, throat, and facial muscles should be performed 5 times daily (see pages 182–184).
- Gargle for 5 minutes twice daily.

Improving your general fitness levels with regular aerobic activity can help reduce the symptoms of sleep apnea.

sleep apnea directly, even without loss of weight. Exercise has also been shown to have positive effects generally on depression and self-rated sleep quality, although for people suffering from sleep disorders, the exercise must be properly timed. Body temperatures rise during exercise and take as long as six hours to begin to drop. Cooler body temperatures are associated with the onset of sleep, so it's important to allow the body time to cool down before sleep.

Exercises to reduce snoring

These throat and tongue exercises stretch and contract the palate and the muscles and tissues in the throat. Conditioned muscles are less likely to make the involuntary movements that cause snoring.

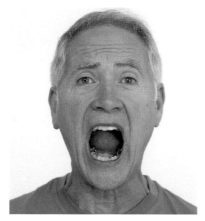

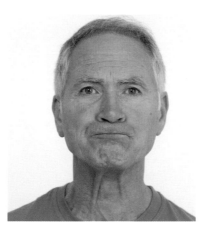

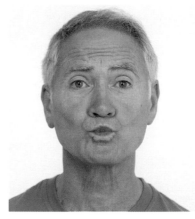

1. *Open your mouth as wide as you can as if you are yawning hugely.*

2. *Then shut your mouth as tightly as you can.*

3. *Pucker up your lips as if you are about to blow a kiss.*

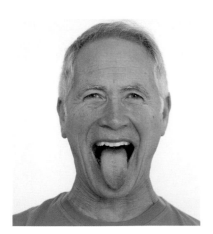

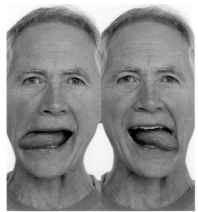

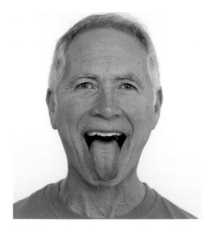

7. *Stick out your tongue. Don't let it waggle around.*

8. *Stick out your tongue again, but this time slide it to each corner of your mouth and keep it there for 10 seconds.*

9. *Stick out your tongue and extend it downward as if you are trying to reach your chin.*

Practice these anti-snoring exercises up to 5 times, twice a day, until snoring is no longer a problem. It takes about 10–15 minutes to do them. Hold each of the positions for 10 seconds and then relax.

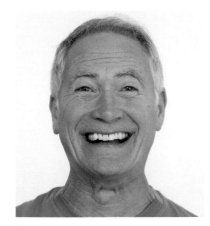

4. *Stretch your lips into a broad, exaggerated smile.*

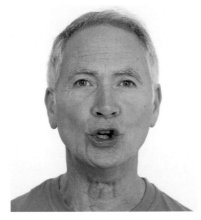

5. *Open your mouth wide and pucker your lips without closing your jaws.*

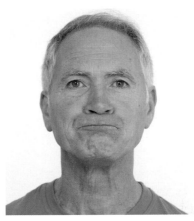

6. *Press your lips tightly together.*

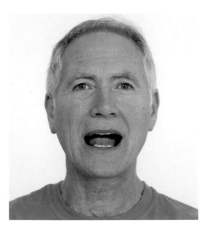

10. *Stick out your tongue and then flick it in and out of your mouth repeatedly as rapidly as possible.*

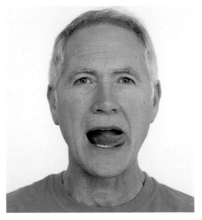

11. *Make the same rapid flicking motion with your tongue, but this time from side to side.*

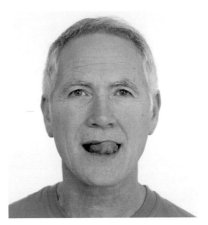

12. *Move the tongue around the lips in a circling motion.*

A workout for the tongue and soft palate

Exercises originally developed for the treatment of speech difficulties have been shown to reduce the severity and symptoms of obstructive sleep apnea significantly. Exercises that raise and lower the soft palate in the roof of the mouth increase the palate's muscle tone. Tongue exercises also increase muscle tone. A strong tongue and soft palate are less likely to collapse into the airway and cause apnea during sleep. Perform each exercise 5–10 times, resting between movements. You will need a straw and a teaspoon.

1. Lightly anchor your tongue between your teeth. Swallow 5 times.

2. Run your tongue around the inside of your mouth and push it between your lips, up around the outside of your teeth, over the roof of your mouth, and down on the base of your mouth. Do this for 10 seconds.

3. Repeat la-la-la-la-la for around 10 seconds, feeling the tip of your tongue curl up to touch just behind your top teeth. Do this 5 times.

4. Work out the back of the tongue by repeating kuh kee kah—kuh kee kah—kuh kee kah, guh gee gah—guh gee gah—guh gee gah, kuh tah kah—kuh tah kah—kuh tah kah, kuh guh kee—kuh guh kee—kuh guh kee. Repeat this sequence 5 times.

5. Place a teaspoon on the palate, behind the front teeth. Elevate the back of the tongue until it touches the edge of the spoon. Press the back of the tongue in place for 3 seconds then relax. Repeat 5 times.

6. Puff air into your cheeks and breathe in and out of your nose. Press a finger against your inflated cheeks. Remember to keep your lips firmly together. Do not allow the air to escape through your mouth or nose. Hold for 10 seconds.

7. Puff up your right cheek. Hold for 5 seconds. Puff up your left cheek. Hold for 5 seconds.

8. Blow out through a straw with your finger over the end. Keep blowing for 5 seconds.

9. Suck a small amount of liquid up through a straw and transfer it to another container, without losing any.

10. Hum with the lips pressed together. Stop humming. Puff out your cheeks. Repeat "p" as you release the air through your teeth.

11. Repeat the hum. Stop humming and puff out your cheeks. As you release air say kuh kee kah—kuh kee kah—kuh kee kah, guh gee gah—guh gee gah—guh gee gah, kuh tah kah—kuh tah kah—kuh tah kah, kuh guh kee—kuh guh kee—kuh guh kee.

12. Practice saying "ssss" without allowing any air to come out through your nose.

13. Make 5 "ah" sounds. Pause between each one.

Chapter 11

Women's Health

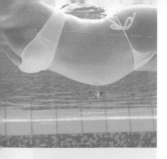

Pregnancy

BEST MOVES

walking

swimming

aqua aerobics

stationary cycling

Pilates

yoga

pelvic-floor exercises

tai chi

Low to moderate levels of exercise while you are pregnant will greatly benefit you and your baby. Low-impact activities, such as walking and aqua aerobics, are a benign way to build or maintain your fitness, but avoid contact sports, high-impact exercise that stresses joints, abdominal muscles, and back muscles, and any activity that puts you at risk of falling, including horseback riding, surfing, waterskiing, and gymnastics. You should also avoid exercising in extreme heat, at high altitude, and in deep water. Keep your heart rate under 140 beats per minute while exercising and avoid overheating, especially in your first trimester.

Inevitably, you will need to modify your exercise regimen to allow for the changes happening in your body as your pregnancy progresses. Hormones produced during pregnancy to soften the body's ligaments in preparation for childbirth can cause joint instability and lower back pain, which is in turn exacerbated by the forward pull of the growing baby. As the baby grows larger, pressure on the diaphragm can cause heartburn and breathlessness. The action of the smooth muscle of the intestines slows down, often causing constipation. The process of childbirth itself weakens the pelvic-floor muscles, which can cause stress incontinence. In the third trimester, you may find it safer

and more comfortable to switch to non-weight bearing exercises, such as swimming and stationary cycling. Even just floating in the water can be beneficial for a pregnant woman carrying the added weight of a baby.

Always seek advice from your doctor regarding any exercise taken during your pregnancy. Special medical considerations may have to be taken into account if you have a history of preterm labor, severe high blood pressure, heart disease, lung disease, severe diabetes, thyroid disease, seizure disorder, or placenta previa, a condition that can cause excessive bleeding before and during pregnancy.

If you have an established running routine, or are already practicing yoga, you can probably continue with it, although hormone-induced hypermobility in the joints, along with added weight stresses in the back and a shift in the body's center of gravity, can have implications for your usual practice. Modify your program as your pregnancy advances, according to how you feel and what your doctor recommends.

During your pregnancy, don't begin any exercise that you have not done before without being properly instructed in a setting where you can receive individual attention. Do not attempt new exercises on your own until a professional has assessed your ability, and you feel comfortable and confident in doing them. Attend yoga, tai chi, or Pilates classes only where the instructor is willing to give you enough one-to-one attention to enable you to modify postures.

Why exercise helps

Not only do women benefit from exercise in pregnancy, but their unborn babies do, too. A recent study found that there were significantly lower heart rates among fetuses that had been exposed to maternal exercise. This study suggests that a mother who exercises may not only be imparting health benefits to her own heart, but to her developing baby's heart as well.

Exercising during pregnancy boosts energy levels, improves general wellbeing, and reduces the likelihood of developing gestational diabetes. It also eases side effects, such as back pain, headaches, fatigue, swelling, varicose veins, and constipation, and lowers maternal blood pressure. Another benefit is that exercise helps to develop the stamina needed to deliver a baby, as well as reducing both the length of labor and the time it takes to recover from giving birth, and a woman who has exercised during pregnancy will find it easier to lose weight after the baby is born. Studies have shown that the risk of premature birth is reduced by about 50 percent by exercising during pregnancy.

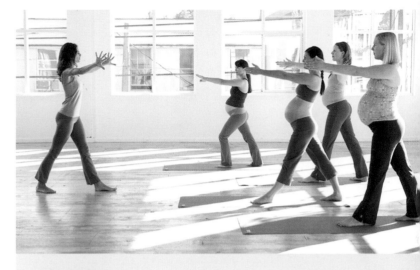

HOW OFTEN?

- **The American College of Obstetricians recommends 30 minutes or more of moderate exercise 3–4 times per week for pregnant women to stay in shape and maintain energy.**
- **In addition, aim to do 3 sets of pelvic-floor exercises, with 10 fast and 10 slow repetitions, per day. Listen to your body. Stop exercising if you have any vaginal bleeding, dizziness, faintness, shortness of breath, contractions, or nauseous feelings. You will also need to adjust the duration of your exercise sessions according to where you are in your pregnancy. Many women experience intense fatigue in their first trimester, as well as nausea, and will need to keep their fitness routines short.**

Above: *Regular exercise in a pregnancy class may suit those in their second trimester, when energy levels are higher. By the time you reach your eighth month, your need for oxygen will have increased by around 10 percent.*

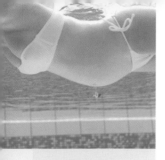

Pregnancy continued

Seek advice from your doctor regarding your exercise program during pregnancy.

Pelvic-floor exercises

During pregnancy, strengthening the perineal muscles, which surround the neck of the bladder and the vagina, can help you to develop the ability to control your muscles during labor and delivery. Toning all of these muscles will also minimize two common problems that arise during pregnancy and sometimes continue afterwards—hemorrhoids and stress incontinence (the involuntary leakage of urine when running, sneezing, or laughing hard).

Perform pelvic-floor exercises by alternately squeezing then releasing the muscles of the perineum. You can strengthen the bladder sphincter itself by tightening, then relaxing, the sphincter. When urinating, stop and start the flow. Contract hard for a second, then release completely. Do this about 10 times in a row, then gradually work your way up to doing 20 sets of 10. (See page 170 for more pelvic-floor exercises.)

Swimming and water exercise

Water provides a weightless environment in which to workout. This is especially beneficial during pregnancy as joints, muscles, and ligaments become susceptible to injury. Increased levels of the hormone progesterone cause them to soften and become overly flexible. Considered the safest exercise for pregnant women, swimming also offers cardiovascular benefits without the risk of overheating. A Brazilian study found that women who do aqua aerobics during pregnancy have easier deliveries and need less pain-relief medication during labor. Healthy pregnant women should be able to continue a regular swimming and water exercise program for the full nine months—avoid scuba diving and waterskiing, though!

Walking

Walking is kinder to your knees than running and can be easily worked into your schedule. Start slowly and be sure to stretch well before you begin. Set realistic goals and wear good shoes to decrease the risk of falling and pressure on your feet.

Running

Your level of fitness when you become pregnant will affect the amount of running your body can handle. If you established a solid running routine before pregnancy, you should be able to continue until running no longer feels comfortable, which generally happens in the seventh month. However, if you did not run before pregnancy, be sure to speak to your doctor before you begin a running program. In any case, if you run, make sure you are well hydrated and avoid overheating.

Cycling

The bike supports your weight, so there is not much stress on your body and that can make cycling a comfortable workout for a pregnant woman. However, your shifting center of gravity puts you at an increased risk of falling, so from the second trimester onward, limit your cycling to a stationary bike.

Yoga

Most forms of yoga will be safe for you and your baby through all three trimesters, as long as they are not excessively rigorous. If possible, go to a yoga class that is especially for pregnant women. Avoid lying flat on your back for extended periods beyond your second trimester, or lying with your feet over your shoulders, and avoid abdominal crunches and curls. Try not to overstretch. Don't do Bikram yoga—it is too overheating for pregnancy.

Tai chi

Tai chi is done standing up with the focus on a strong back and legs. It promotes good posture and reduces back pain, and can help women avoid many of the circulatory problems experienced during pregnancy, such as varicose veins and deep vein thrombosis. Tai chi's leg actions help blood and lymph to circulate from the lower limbs back to the heart.

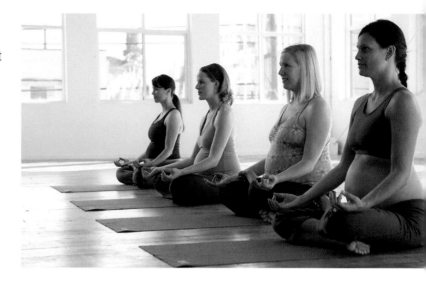

Pilates

Practicing Pilates through pregnancy can help you tone your core (including pelvic-floor muscles), train your internal muscles to be strong yet flexible, and help minimize the back and hip ache that many pregnant women experience. You will need to be assessed by a Pilates instructor to see if you can contract your pelvic floor or deep abdominal muscles effectively. Very basic Pilates exercises are designed to achieve this. Pilates exercises are also beneficial after the baby has been born (see pages 190–191).

Practicing yoga during pregnancy is great for relaxation and muscle tone.

189

Pilates postnatal exercises

SPINE CURLS mobilize the spine and hips, and strengthen the back, abdominals, buttocks, and backs of the legs.

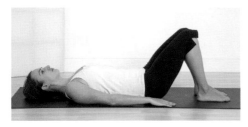 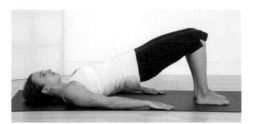

3. Breathe out as you roll the spine back down, slowly and evenly through each section. Breathe in as you release the pelvis back to the start position.

1. Start by lying on your back, with your knees raised and arms down by your sides. Breathe in to prepare.

2. Breathe out as you curl your pelvis downward, pressing the lower back on the floor before peeling bone by bone off the mat. Roll to the tips of the shoulder blades. Breathe in and hold, keeping the shoulders wide and relaxed, weight equal on both feet. Lift the buttocks to prevent the back arching.

SPINE CURLS WITH LEG EXTENSION

1. At the top of the spine curl position, breathe in to prepare and as you breathe out extend one leg, keeping the knees level. Try to avoid any movement in the hips.

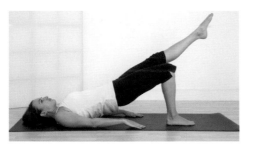

2. Breathe in when you lower the foot, and breathe out when extending the other leg. Keep the buttocks lifted and torso long—try not to allow the spine to arch. Breathe in to lower the foot, and breathe out to roll the spine back to the floor, vertebra by vertebra. Repeat up to 5 times with each leg.

OYSTER/CLAMS mobilize hips and strengthen buttocks and knee joints.

1. Lie on your side, with shoulders, hips, knees, and ankles stacked. Head, spine, and bottom should be in line with the back of the mat. Lengthen your lower arm underneath your

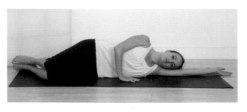 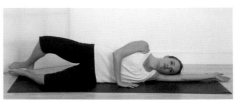

head, in line with your spine. Place your top hand on the mat in front of your ribcage, bending the elbow. Bend both knees and draw your feet back so they are in line with your bottom.

2. Breathe in to prepare. As you breathe out, open your top knee, keeping the feet together. Only open the leg as far as you can without disturbing the position of the pelvis—do not allow it to tip back. Keep your chest open. Breathe in and bring the leg down slowly. Repeat 5 times, then repeat on the other side.

SIDE-LYING CIRCLES mobilize and strengthen hips and core.

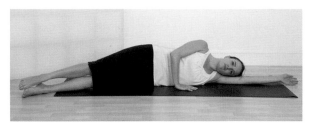

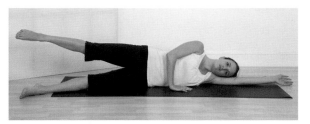

1. *Lie on your side in a straight line, lower arm extended along the floor and top arm, palm down, on the mat in front of your ribcage. Carry both legs forward, hinging from the hip, so that they are slightly in front of the body. Make sure the waist is long and the chest is open. Breathe in to prepare, and as you breathe out, lift and extend the top leg just higher than hip height, with toes softly pointed. Keep your stomach firm to help you balance.*

2. *Breathe out and circle the leg. The circle should be about the size of a football. Keep the circle even and the legs parallel. Breathe in to repeat. Repeat up to 5 times in one direction, then circle the leg in the opposite direction. Control any wobbling, keeping your stomach lifted for support, and lengthen the underneath leg for balance. Lower with an inbreath, and repeat on the other side.*

SIDE-LYING LIFTS tone outer thighs and strengthen obliques and core.

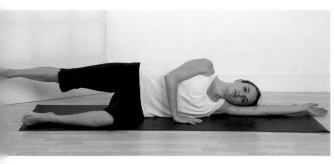

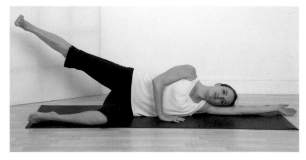

1. *Lie on your side in a straight line, lower arm extended along the floor and top arm on the mat, palm down, in front of the ribcage. Bend your knees as if sitting in a chair. Keep the waist long and stomach lifted. Breathe in to prepare. Exhale and extend the top leg, in line with the body, at hip height. Flex the foot. Keep ribs soft and stomach strong so the back does not arch. Keep the leg parallel to the ground, kneecap forward.*

2. *Breathe out and slowly lift the leg as far as you can while keeping your waist long on both sides (do not allow the waist to sag toward the floor) and the pelvis still. Think about keeping the leg long, pressing through the heel—long waist, long leg. Keep the upper body open. Raise and lower your leg 10 times, exhale to lift, inhale to lower. Bend the top leg down, and repeat on the other side.*

THE CAT develops mobility in the spine and strengthens the abdominals.

1. *Start on all fours, hands directly underneath the shoulders, and knees directly underneath the hips. Lengthen through the spine. Keep the neck long and do not allow the head to drop. Breathe in to prepare.*

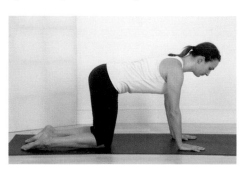

2. *Breathe out, lift the tummy and roll the pelvis underneath you, rounding the lower back. Continue, allowing your upper body to round gradually, followed by your neck, and finally tuck the chin toward the chest and nod the head slightly forward. Keep the abdominals engaged. Breathe in wide to the lower ribcage to hold the position. Breathe out as your start to unfurl the spine, sending the tailbone away from the crown of the head. Lengthen the spine back to the start position, neck long. Repeat up to 10 times.*

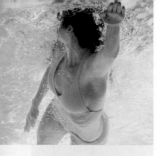

BEST MOVES

resistance
training

brisk walking

cycling

swimming

Pilates

yoga

tai chi

Menopause

Menopause, the ending of a woman's menstrual periods and reproductive capacity, occurs on average around the age of 52. The transition into menopause is called perimenopause and its duration varies widely from a few months to years. Menstruation typically becomes more unpredictable during perimenopause, and fluctuating symptoms include hot flashes, chills, vaginal dryness, breast tenderness, sleep disruptions, headaches, palpitations, and mood swings. Most of these symptoms, and body changes such as loss of muscle tone, thinning hair, drier skin, and weight gain, are related to declining levels of the hormone estrogen. A woman is considered to have reached menopause once 12 months have passed since her last period. At that point, her ovaries no longer release eggs and production of estrogen is much reduced. Although menopause is not a medical event, it can be a turbulent time for many women, both physically and emotionally.

Why exercise helps
Regular aerobic exercise increases estrogen levels, which helps to provide relief from hot flashes and other symptoms of menopause, and resistance training builds muscle. A woman can lose as much as 30 percent of total muscle mass between the ages of 50 and 80. Resistance training strengthens muscles and reduces bone loss and fractures, which become more common as estrogen levels fall. Pilates, tai chi, and yoga help to loosen up stiff limbs by improving range of motion and joint flexibility. The calming, mood-balancing benefits of yoga and tai chi are helpful to women whose hormonal levels and body chemistry may be fluctuating rapidly.

Physically active postmenopausal women are less likely than inactive women to develop a complex of related disorders known as metabolic syndrome, which often starts at menopause. The syndrome causes excessive weight gain, particularly around the middle, high cholesterol levels, higher blood sugar, and increased resistance to the hormone insulin. Postmenopausal women who exercise regularly are about half as likely to develop diabetes as women who are sedentary. If extra weight is carried into the menopause years, the risk of breast cancer rises. Exercise, especially in the morning, gets lymphatic and circulatory systems moving and activates the liver to process waste more efficiently, which encourages a healthy immune system.

Sex
According to Dr June Reinisch, former director of the Kinsey Institute at Indiana University, postmenopausal women who regularly orgasm may have a reduced chance of contracting urinary tract or vaginal infections. She believes that

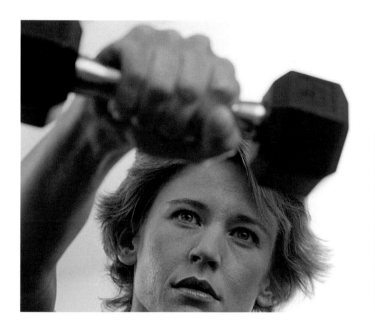

HOW OFTEN?
- Aim to work out for an hour at least 4 or 5 days per week, using a balanced routine of resistance training combined with aerobic and flexibility training. For example: resistance training 2–3 times per week alternating with aerobic exercise and at least one session each week of flexibility training. Stretches should be done before and after each resistance or aerobic session. You might want to work with a personal trainer to get started, or find aerobic, strength training, and flexibility classes specifically for beginners.

regular sexual activity provides continuous lubrication of the vaginal area and counteracts the dryness that may be conducive to infection. Accumulating evidence indicates sex may have some therapeutic value for a number of menopause symptoms.

Skin

Many women feel dispirited about their appearance as they come to terms with signs of aging. Exercise releases endorphins that reduce stress and boost self-esteem. These feel-good hormones will do your skin a favor, too. When you are stressed, your brain releases insulin, cortisol, and other "anxiety" hormones that age the skin. Collagen is a type of protein that works with elastin to keep your skin looking firm and smooth, but stress hormones switch on enzymes that break down collagen and cause wrinkles. Exercise keeps stress hormones at bay and expands blood vessels so that more oxygen and nutrients become available to promote collagen production.

As you grow older, rising blood sugar levels produce glucosepane, which acts on collagen to make it tougher and less flexible. By keeping your blood sugar levels in check, exercise reduces the production of glucosepane, boosting the quality of the collagen in your tissues. It also gives your skin a healthy glow when you sweat, which unclogs pores and clarifies the complexion.

Above: *Resistance training with weights helps build muscle mass and bone density. Strong bones guard against osteoporosis.*

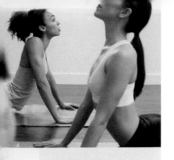

Menstruation

BEST MOVES
brisk walking
running
swimming
cycling
dancing
yoga
Pilates

A woman's menstrual cycle consists of four phases that last approximately 28 days and are programed by the hormones estrogen and progesterone. These hormones also cause changes in mood and other physical symptoms. The menstrual phase begins on the first day of a period, when bleeding indicates that the lining of the uterus is being shed, and lasts for around four days. The follicular phase comes next and lasts from approximately day five through to day 13. During this stage, menstruation lightens and ovarian follicles begin to ripen. On day 14, approximately, ovulation occurs, when a follicle releases an egg.

The remaining days of the 28-day cycle are known as the luteal phase. During this phase, increased estrogen and progesterone create changes in the lining of the uterus that prepare it to accept an embryo. If conception does not occur, estrogen and progesterone levels decline, and the lining of the uterus, called the endometrial lining, begins to shed as menstrual bleeding.

During the end part of this luteal phase many women experience bloating, cramps, anxiety, depression, food cravings, fatigue, backache, and headaches. The sharp drop in hormone levels that occurs in the last week before a period begins causes physical and emotional symptoms that are known as premenstrual syndrome (PMS) or premenstrual tension (PMT).

Why exercise helps

Women who exercise regularly experience less premenstrual tension, less menstrual discomfort, shorter periods, and less bleeding. Exercise also strengthens the pelvic floor, so reproductive organs are better supported.

Aerobic exercise during your period helps decrease the pain of cramps by increasing blood flow, which relaxes muscles in the lower abdomen, back,

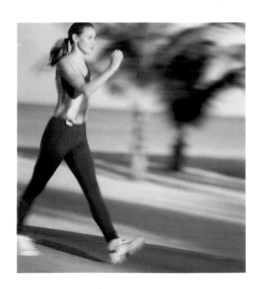

Brisk walking helps ease the symptoms of premenstrual tension, and can also mean lighter periods.

and thighs, and releases endorphins (the body's natural painkillers), which improve and stabilize mood. Endorphins help to burn prostaglandins, the chemicals released during menstruation that cause muscle contractions. Exercise that works up a sweat helps to dissipate bloating and fluid retention.

Most women find that their energy levels rise in the second half of their cycle, after ovulation. An Australian study found that exercising after ovulation, compared with exercising in the first week of the menstrual cycle, also burns more fat. In the early part of the menstrual cycle, when estrogen and progesterone are low, levels of waste products, such as blood lactate, are higher and your muscles feel the "burn" more quickly. As levels of these hormones rise in the second half of the cycle, your metabolism becomes more efficient at burning fat and you generally feel able to push yourself harder physically.

Yoga poses that improve pelvic blood flow can give considerable relief from pelvic pain and discomfort. Some schools of yoga advise women not to do upside-down poses while menstruating, because they can lead to vascular congestion—more blood enters the uterus via the arteries than can be carried away by the veins, which may increase menstrual bleeding. Not all yoga systems follow this rule and it's up

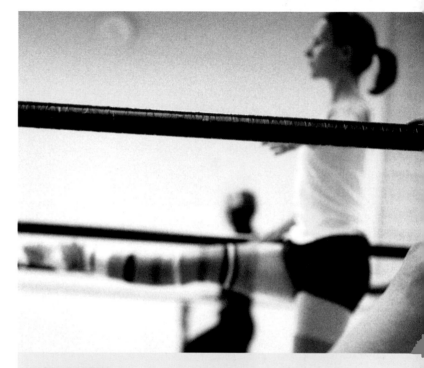

HOW OFTEN?

- Do some aerobic exercise every second day for up to 60 minutes at a time. When stress aggravates period pain or PMS, undertaking slow, repetitive, and rhythmic distance exercise, such as walking, cycling, or swimming, at a moderate pace for about an hour will have a calming effect as well as improving stamina.
- Listen to your body and adapt your training regimen or activity levels according to how you feel across your menstrual cycle. Many women report an improvement in PMS if they exercise during the week leading up to their period.
- If you are suffering from menstrual cramps that are too painful to allow you to exercise, take a few days off from your exercise schedule, or focus on a calming physical activity, such as restorative yoga or qigong.

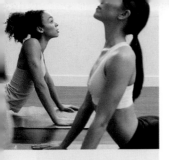

Endorphins help to burn prostaglandins, the chemicals released during menstruation that cause muscle contractions.

Menstruation continued

to individual women to see how they feel about practicing inversions during their periods.

Pilates and endometriosis

Endometriosis is a condition in which tissue similar to the lining of the uterus grows outside of the uterus, usually in the abdomen. Women with endometriosis can suffer pelvic pain at any time during their monthly cycle. Menstrual bleeding can be very painful. The pain of endometriosis often makes women stay away from physical activity, but lack of exercise weakens the muscles, deconditions the body, and undermines overall health. Pilates is a very gentle set of exercises, designed to strengthen abdominal and back

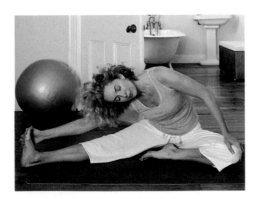

Practicing Pilates builds strong core muscles and helps ease the pain of endometriosis.

Yoga poses that are beneficial for menstruation:

Forward bends are calming poses that compress the lower abdomen and pelvis, which gives relief from cramps and reduces heavy bleeding.

Standing poses using a wall or a chair for support help relieve the backache associated with menstruation.

Twists are helpful for cramps and backache.

muscles, and women with endometriosis may find them helpful in managing their condition and reducing levels of pain.

Exercise-induced amenorrhea

Some women are concerned about the role exercise has to play in causing irregular periods or stopping the menstrual cycle completely. This condition, known as exercise-induced amenorrhea, applies only to women who regularly undertake vigorous, prolonged exercise, such as running more than 25 miles (40km) per week. Women training at this intensity lose significant amounts of body fat and, since fat cells are essential for hormone production, the menstrual cycle becomes disrupted. Exercise-induced amenorrhea is not an issue for women who exercise for an hour a day.

Chapter 12

Aging

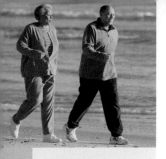

Aging

BEST MOVES

walking

swimming

aqua aerobics

resistance training

gardening

dancing

Pilates

yoga

qigong

tai chi

We know that regular exercise can help prevent or control conditions commonly associated with the aging process, such as high blood pressure, stroke, heart disease, diabetes, weight gain, osteoporosis, chronic obstructive pulmonary disease, constipation, incontinence, and arthritis. Now research has shown that exercise can actually make your DNA younger and healthier. One of the factors in aging is the length of the telomeres, the protective ends of your chromosomes. As you age, your telomeres shrink, which increases the risk of disease. Researchers who compared exercise habits and telomere length in identical twins were able to prove that lifestyle choices, such as physical activity, really do have an effect on longevity. Those who exercised vigorously for at least three hours each week had longer telomeres and their biological age was reckoned to be nine years younger than those of the same chronological age who did no exercise.

Not only is exercising good for physical wellbeing, it's good for the brain, too. Older adults who exercise regularly are likely to experience improvements in memory and other areas of cognitive function. Researchers at the University of Illinois found that even relatively short exercise sessions can restore some of the losses in brain volume that come with aging. Other studies have suggested that exercise may cause a reduction of the vascular disease associated with dementia.

Much of the age-related loss of fitness we take for granted is due to inactivity rather than age alone. Embarking on a routine of physical fitness later in life will show benefits almost straightaway. Strength-training exercise, in particular, stimulates the body to produce human-growth hormone, the "Fountain of Youth" that

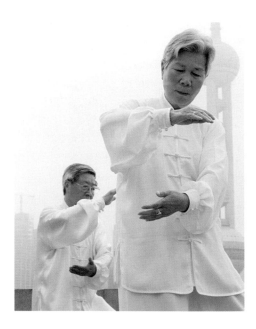

Practicing tai chi helps to develop a strong sense of balance.

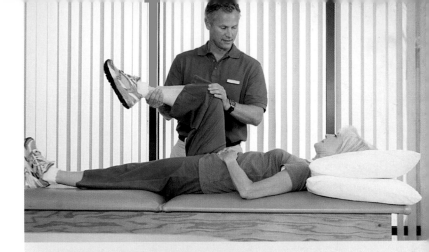

rejuvenates aging cells and helps build muscle, burn body fat, and boost capacity for endurance. Endurance abilities can actually improve with age, as is witnessed by the number of older runners who do well in ultramarathons, where staying power is more effective than speed.

Apart from specific health gains, one of the most compelling reasons to stay fit in later life is the ability to maintain independence. A 65-year-old who exercises regularly and eats a healthy diet can expect to live without any disabilities until age 83 or longer.

Why exercise helps

Exercise slows down the aging process and relieves some of the problems that are commonly associated with getting older, including insomnia, back and joint pain, stress, and tension. Physical activity will counter the energy drain associated with disability and depression. The optimal exercise program for health and longevity combines resistance training for the muscles, cardiovascular (aerobic) workouts for the heart, and flexibility and stretching exercises for the joints.

Resistance training

Using free weights, exercise machines, or elastic bands, resistance training builds and strengthens muscles and

HOW OFTEN?

- At least 3 hours of combined resistance training, aerobic exercise, and flexibility workouts each week are recommended by the American National Institute on Aging. Anything you do to move around and use your body will be good for you, even if it is just walking for 10 minutes each day. Gradually integrate more physical activity into your week.
- A tai chi or yoga class once or twice a week will do wonders for your sense of balance, your flexibility, and your peace of mind.
- One or two 30-minute weight-training sessions per week will keep muscles strong. Use free weights, elastic bands, or machines at your local fitness center, or do aqua aerobics at your local pool. As you build up your stamina, you may be able to do longer gym sessions of up to 60 minutes 2 or 3 times per week, combining resistance training and aerobic workouts. Don't forget to warm up for 10 minutes before you begin.
- Ask a trainer at the gym or fitness center to show you how to do isolated (one-joint) strength-training exercises, such as a bicep curl or chest fly, for each major muscle group. After completing 3 sets of 12 repetitions for each muscle group, move on to 20 minutes of aerobic work on a stationary cycle or treadmill, then cool down with stretches for 10 minutes. Maintain enthusiasm by mixing up the types of exercise you do.
- You don't have to follow the same routine every day. If you find yourself becoming a little bored, find a new form of physical activity to pique your interest.

Above: *Have a trainer assess your flexibility and design a program of stretches for you.*

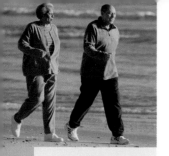

Aging continued

Exercise slows down the aging process and relieves some of the problems that are commonly associated with getting older, including insomnia, back and joint pain, stress, and tension.

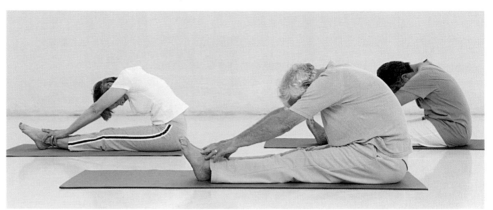

increases bone density. This can slow down or even reverse the aging process. Improved muscle strength helps arrest functional decline, allowing older people to carry on with everyday tasks, such as climbing stairs, getting out of chairs, bathing, and doing housework.

Muscle strengthening and balance retraining programs can significantly decrease the risk of falls. After the age of 65, one in three people will fall during normal activities of daily living. Falls in later years often result in wrist and hip fractures, which lead to hospitalizations and loss of independence. Resistance exercise also helps lower moderately high blood pressure while encouraging the metabolism to work faster, an important factor in maintaining a healthy body weight.

It's never too late to start. Numerous studies show that even people in their 80s demonstrate considerable increases

Flexibility exercises have a calming effect on the nervous system. Combine them with resistance training and an aerobic activity for maximum benefit.

in strength and power after beginning moderate resistance training using machines and weights.

Aerobic workouts

There's no getting around the fact that aerobic capacity falls with age, but the longer you continue with any exercise that pumps oxygen into your system and works your lungs and heart—whether it's walking, cycling, swimming, jogging, dancing, or playing tennis—the longer your aerobic capacity will take to decline. A Harvard University study of 72,000 women found that three hours of brisk walking every week cut their risk of heart disease by 40 percent. A similar study of 2,700 elderly men in Hawaii found that those who walked 1½ miles (2.4km) or more per day were half as likely to develop heart trouble as men who seldom walked.

Aqua aerobics is an ideal workout for people with brittle bones, arthritis, and other age-related conditions. Water's cushioning effect protects from injury and fear of injury. Joining an aqua aerobics class has the added benefit of sociability—isolation and loneliness can be issues for older people. In a study of 156 severely depressed men and women over 50, Duke University researchers suggest that 16 weeks of aerobic exercise may be as effective in alleviating the illness as a 16-week regimen of antidepressant drugs.

Flexibility exercises

A wide-ranging analysis of balance studies found that people who practice yoga and tai chi had a significantly better sense of joint position and better reaction times than people of the same age who did not practice such balance-intensive activities. Tai chi, yoga, and Pilates all require slow deliberate movements, trunk rotation, and one-legged stances, and practicing them helps to prevent falls. In addition to improving flexibility and balance, tai chi, yoga, and Pilates improve cardiovascular health, muscle strength, handgrip strength, coordination, and sleep quality.

Qigong, tai chi, and yoga have a calming effect upon the nervous system and are beneficial in the treatment of anxiety, insomnia, and depression. Their gentle approach to mind-body integration makes them well suited to frail people who are coping with chronic pain.

Running at 50+

Running is a brilliant way to stay fit and muscle-toned as you get older, as long as you take care to modify your training routine to take account of the fact that you're not as young as you once were.

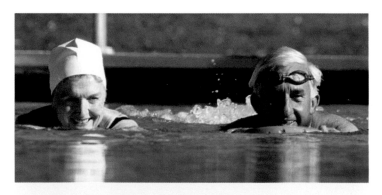

A seven-day training program might look like this
- Day 1: 20 minutes' weight training
- Day 2: 30 minutes' easy run or rest day
- Day 3: 45 minutes' cross train, e.g. swim or tai chi/yoga/stretches
- Day 4: 30 minutes' weight training
- Day 5: 30 minutes' interval workout
- Day 6: rest day
- Day 7: 60 minutes' slow jog

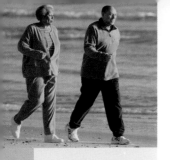

A wide-ranging analysis of balance studies found that people who practice yoga and tai chi had a significantly better sense of joint position and better reaction times than people of the same age who did not practice such balance-intensive activities.

Aging continued

Of course, you should check with your doctor, but as long as you don't have any pre-existing health issues that preclude it, you can successfully take up running in your later years. Before you start, read everything you can about training for older runners and seek advice from a running coach at your local gym.

Your training program will begin with an exercise in patience. Older beginners need to walk before they run. It may take weeks of walking before you feel fit and confident enough to add some very slow, occasional running to your walks—for example, doing 20-minute sessions that alternate 30 seconds of running with three minutes of walking. Gradually, you will be able to increase the amount of time spent running and decrease the time spent walking. This slow transition will help prevent injuries and build strength and endurance in the muscles. You might take another few weeks of combined walk/run sessions before you find yourself mostly running. Even then, if you feel you need to take a break and walk—then walk. The idea is to keep safe from injury so that you can continue running right into your 70s and even 80s. You want to be able to enjoy the incredible buzz that comes from running for as long as possible.

Try to run one high-intensity session each week, alternating sprints with recovery intervals—for example, sprint

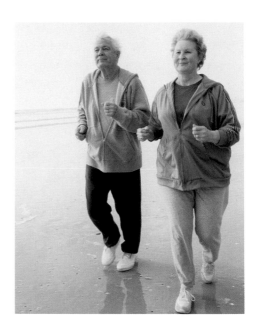

It is possible to enjoy the benefits of running far into your senior years—providing you take it slowly to start with and rest when you need to.

for 60 to 90 seconds, followed by five minutes of easy jogging. Older runners take longer to recover, so don't set fierce goals for yourself. If your body wants to rest, let it rest.

As we age, rest is critical for injury prevention. Don't run every day, and practice several other activities as well, such as light weight lifting, stretching, swimming, or cycling, to keep strong and limber and aid recovery. Muscle strength helps to maintain running speed as we age.

Balance exercises

After the age of 65, the risk of falling increases significantly; in fact, it becomes the number-one threat to the health and independence of older people. Exercise programs, especially those that include balance training, have been widely recognized by experts in older people's health as an effective means of reducing falls.

KNEE RAISES help to build strength in thighs and hip flexors.

1. *Stand beside a chair, your right side next to its back.*

2. *Place your right hand on the back of the chair. Put your weight on your inside (right) leg, keeping your knee soft and slightly bent.*

3. *Take a deep breath. As you exhale, bend and raise your left knee. Stand tall with stomach muscles engaged. Resist the urge to bend at the waist or hips as you do this balancing move. Inhale and hold the knee raise for 3 seconds while using the chair for support.*

4. *With an exhalation, return your leg back to the floor. Repeat several times and then switch legs.*

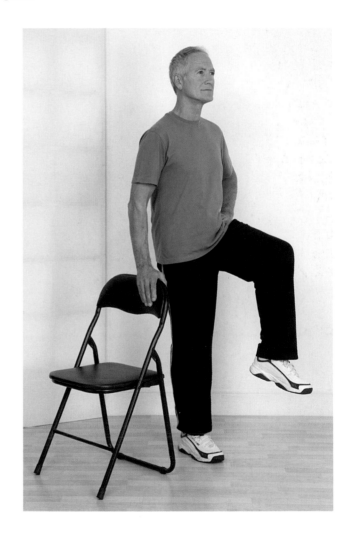

Balance exercises continued

SIDE LEG RAISES help to build strength in legs and hip flexors.

1. Stand behind the chair, right side on. Keep your back straight. Place your feet flat on the floor and slightly apart. Hold on to the back of the chair.

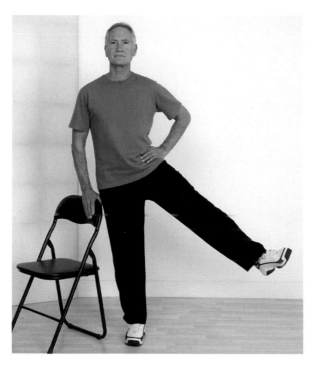

2. Take a deep breath and as you exhale slowly lift your left leg off the floor to the side. Keep both legs straight and your toes pointed forward. Inhale and hold this pose for a few seconds. As you exhale return to the starting position. Repeat this several times, alternating legs.

HIP EXTENSIONS help to build strength in lower back, hips, and buttocks.

1. Stand facing the back of the chair with your feet flat on the floor and slightly less than shoulder-width apart. Slowly lift one leg straight back, keeping the leg and knee straight. Keep your back straight as you do this move.

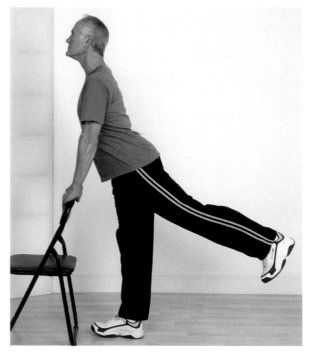

2. Hold the pose for a second and then slowly return your leg to the starting position. Repeat this several times and then switch legs.

Chapter 13

Cancer Prevention

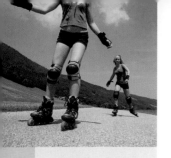

Cancer prevention

BEST MOVES

power walking

running

cycling

skiing

rollerblading

surfing

climbing

kickboxing

capoeira

tae bo

ashtanga yoga

martial arts

dancing

spinning

kickfit

boxing

step aerobics

bootcamp

Our bodies are made up of hundreds of different types of cells, which behave according to instructions they receive from the genetic codes stored in their nuclei. Cancer occurs when a mutation in the codes causes a cell to respond to instructions that are wrong. The cell begins dividing uncontrollably and with every division the erroneous instruction is compounded. The fast-multiplying cells form a lump, or tumor. Sometimes

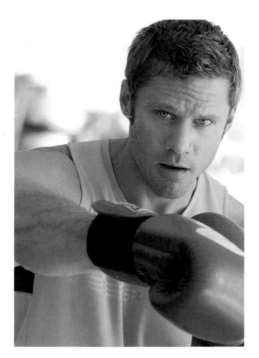

Physical movement is needed to disperse toxins from our bodies. Breaking sweat reduces cancer risk.

the tumor is benign, which means it will not invade neighboring tissues and organs. However, if the tumor is malignant, or cancerous, it will spread beyond its original site and cause damage to tissues that is potentially fatal. Genetic predisposition, environmental circumstances, and lifestyle choices all influence a person's risk of contracting cancer.

Some human cancers are linked to pre-existing viral infections, among them liver cancer (caused by the hepatitis B and C viruses), cervical cancer (from human papillomavirus), cancers of the genital and anal area, T-cell leukemia, and lymphomas caused by the Epstein–Barr virus. This doesn't mean that these cancers can be caught like a cold or flu. It means that a pre-existing virus can cause genetic alterations to cells that make them more likely to become cancerous. Most types of cancer become more common as people age because the longer we live, the more time there is for genetic mistakes to take place in our cells.

Why exercise helps

Physical activity, a balanced diet, healthy body weight, and not smoking are factors that have been proven in countless studies to be modifiable cancer risk factors. The influence of exercise on hormone levels, immune

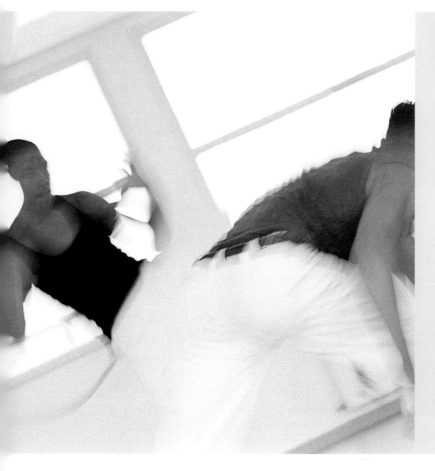

HOW OFTEN?
- Cancer experts recommend that men and women undertake at least 30 minutes of dedicated exercise on at least 5 days per week, above and beyond their usual activities.
- Researchers say that even moderate amounts of exercise protect against colon cancer.
- Other investigations have concluded that the more vigorously active you are, the greater the cancer-prevention benefits.
- A study in Finland found that subjects who did intense aerobic exercise for at least 30 minutes per day halved their risk of dying of cancer compared with those who exercised less. Intense aerobic exercise was measured at 5.2 MET (metabolic units of oxygen consumption).

function, and body weight plays an important role in preventing many cancers. Exercise helps to boost the immune systems of people at genetic risk of contracting virally transmitted cancers. White blood cells in our immune system protect the body by fighting off infections and diseases. These defender cells are transferred around the body by the lymphatic system. Unlike blood, which is pumped by the heart, the lymphatic system does not have its own pumping mechanism. Physical movement is needed to assist lymph in its drainage and cleansing work.

The World Cancer Research Fund recommends that men and women aim to be as lean as possible without becoming underweight. Overweight

Above: *Regular aerobic activity helps prevent cancer by keeping you lean.*

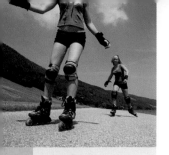

Cancer prevention continued

CANCER PREVENTION

Exercise helps to boost the immune systems of people at genetic risk of contracting virally transmitted cancers.

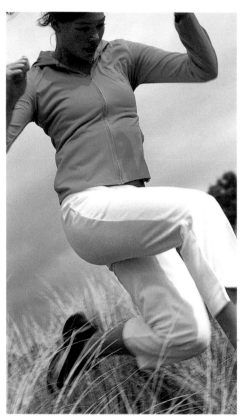

An influential recent study says that high-intensity exercise is best for lowering the risk of contracting cancer, particularly lung and gastrointestinal cancers.

women have raised levels of the hormone estrogen in their blood. That puts them at risk of cancers of the breast and reproductive system, which are sensitive to estrogen. In a Harvard study, women who had been athletes in their teens and early 20s were shown to have a lower lifetime rate of cancer of the breast and of the uterus, ovaries, cervix, and vagina than women who were not athletes. Exercise may have protected them indirectly, by helping them remain lean.

Taking up a regular exercise routine at any age will help. Investigators in a study of more than 30,000 postmenopausal American women found that the risk of developing breast cancer after menopause was lower by about one-third in women who undertook vigorous physical activity compared with women who had generally undertaken little physical exercise in their lives.

An extensive new study by Washington University School of Medicine and Harvard University found that men and women who exercised the most were 24 percent less likely to develop colon cancer than those who exercised the least, no matter what the intensity of the exercise. Physical activity protects against colon cancer, whether it is moderate walking or jogging, biking or swimming, by stimulating the muscle movement of the large intestine. This speeds up the passage of fecal contents and minimizes the amount of time the colon wall is in contact with the dangerous toxins carried in feces. Moderate regular exercise, such as walking for several hours a week, may also help protect men from prostate cancer. Researchers studying men who had a prostate biopsy found that those who were moderately active were significantly less likely to be diagnosed with prostate cancer.

However, an influential recent study from Finland says that high-intensity exercise is best for lowering the risk of contracting cancer and dying from it, particularly lung and gastrointestinal cancers. Investigators at Kuopio and Oulu Universities followed the exercise habits of more than 2,000 men for 17 years and discovered that those who exercised intensely and frequently were much less likely to die of cancer. This was still the case after adjusting for factors such as age, alcohol consumption, smoking, body weight, and calorie intake. The investigators believe the benefits arise from an improved balance between energy expenditure and body mass as well as lower testosterone levels and the reduced amount of time it takes for food

Intensity of exercise measured in MET (see page 207)
- running 10.1
- skiing 9.6
- ball games 6.7
- swimming 5.4
- cycling 5.1
- gymnastics, dancing and weight lifting 5
- gardening 4.3
- walking 4.2

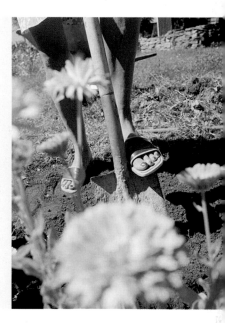

to travel through the bowel. The body's excretory systems are responsible for releasing toxins.

Scientists have not yet been able to ascertain the link between exercise and prevention in many of the more than 200 cancers that have been identified, especially as some cancers can take 20 years or more to produce symptoms.

Chapter 14

Exercise Directory

Aerobics

Regular aerobic exercise strengthens the heart and lungs, helps to lower blood pressure and cholesterol, and burns calories. It stimulates the circulation of lymph and strengthens the immune system. Aerobic exercise raises serotonin levels, triggering the release of endorphins, feel-good hormones that ease stress and anxiety.

The term "aerobics" usually refers to group fitness classes featuring aerobic exercise set to music. An instructor leads participants through a variety of structured movements that are designed to raise the heart rate and stimulate the flow of blood and oxygen. An aerobics class usually lasts from 45 minutes to an hour. The class generally starts with warm-up exercises, including stretches, and gradually revs up to high-intensity exercises that really get your heart working, before easing down with moves that lower the heart rate.

Some aerobics classes are specifically low-impact for people who are not comfortable with movements that put pressure on the joints. Low-impact aerobics stay with exercises that involve keeping at least one foot on the floor at all times. They tend to be suitable for pregnant women, older people, overweight people, and those recovering from injury.

There are many variations of aerobics classes on offer. You can find classes that incorporate moves from boxing, martial arts, dance, and other dynamic disciplines. Step aerobics uses a raised platform or "step" to accelerate and intensify the workout to your lower body. Small free weights are often used in step classes. Pump classes use barbells and free weights to do strength and body conditioning work to music.

Aqua or water aerobics

Aqua aerobics are group aerobic classes that take place in a swimming pool. The classes condition the body, as well as the lungs and heart, and burn calories. An instructor on the side of the pool demonstrates the exercises, and participants, standing chest-high in the water, perform them to music. Workout sessions generally last from 45 minutes to an hour.

Water provides a gentle resistance to movements, which helps to improve strength and muscle tone. It is also buoyant and supports your body while you move, which makes it a safe and comfortable form of exercise, particularly for people who have weight or joint problems, or who are disabled in some way. Being in water is soothing to most people and it therefore has wellbeing as well as health benefits. Aqua aerobics are particularly beneficial and relaxing for pregnant women and people with heart problems, arthritis, back pain, or osteoporosis.

Aquatone

A variation on aqua aerobics, aquatone incorporates strength-building exercises that target specific muscle groups. The class uses the whole pool. Many movements require you to use both arms and legs to travel from one side of the pool to the other.

Boxing for fitness

Fitness boxing classes and circuits at gyms involve boxing training without full-contact body strikes. Fitness boxing is an intense, challenging whole-body workout that improves the cardiovascular system and overall muscle strength, and maximizes calorie burn. Most classes at boxing gyms or health clubs are an hour in length. They consist of a 10-minute warm-up followed by boxing-specific strength and conditioning exercises. Punching techniques are introduced in each session. Then the workout focuses on drills of punch combinations, which require concentration and speed. They last for two- or three-minute rounds, with one-minute recovery periods. The drills are performed in a circuit-training format where you aim punches variously at focus pads, speed bags, and heavy bags. The class ends with a cool-down period.

Fitness boxing is a great activity to vary your exercise regime, and a terrific alternative for serious runners and cyclists wanting to maintain fitness in the winter.

Capoeira

An energetic and graceful Brazilian martial arts technique, capoeira combines combat-style moves, such as kicking and spinning, with dance moves and cartwheels. It developed as a form of martial arts disguised as dance that once allowed Brazilian slaves to train for fighting without detection by their captors. The dance-move "sparring" sessions of capoeira are performed either solo or with a partner. Your butt, quads, and hamstrings get a real workout thanks to multiple repetitions of the ginga—a deep, side-to-side lunge that links one capoeira movement to the next.

Circuit training

Circuit training combines aerobic and resistance training, and targets fat loss, muscle building, and heart-lung fitness. A circuit session starts with walking and stretching and goes on to a series of eight to 15 exercises performed in sequence, each for a couple of minutes only, with a rapid transition from one to the next. For example, pedaling on a bike for three minutes, then doing squats for 30 seconds. A circuit is one round of all prescribed exercises in a program. It can include use of weights, resistance machines, stationary bicycles, treadmills, rowing machines, and exercise balls, and floor exercises. When one circuit is complete, you begin the first exercise again for another round.

Climbing (indoor)

Indoor rock climbing calls for the same fitness, muscle strength, and endurance as the outdoor version. It is an activity that builds upper-body strength, tones the body, builds stamina, and burns calories. Indoor climbing involves ascending from the floor toward the ceiling of an indoor "rock" wall, textured to resemble a cliff face. The climb is made by gripping holds (made of resin) with your hands and feet. The need to find a viable route up the face of the "cliff" provides a satisfying mental challenge. Climbers wear a safety harness to prevent them from falling.

Cycling (outdoor)

Cycling for fitness provides an excellent, low-impact, cardiovascular workout, and improves the body's ability to use oxygen. Pedaling uses the big muscle groups—the quads at the front of the thighs and the hamstrings at the back. Cycling tones the thighs and buttocks, and strengthens the back and abdomen.

The bike needs to be set up to provide a comfortable riding position, and adjusting the saddle is critical. It must be at the right height for you, and the right distance from the handlebars and pedals. For stability, handlebars should be as wide as the shoulders.

Fitness riding can be a solitary activity, but it becomes much more rewarding and sociable if you join a club and ride with a group.

Cycling (indoor)

Indoor cycling workouts have the same physiological benefits as outdoor rides. The main difference between cycling indoors on a stationary bike and outdoors on a real bike is wind resistance. Indoors, the lack of wind makes it easier to spin the wheels at a higher speed, but if you produce the same power, both workouts will be equally beneficial. Indoor cycling, like its outdoor equivalent, will strengthen your heart and improve lung capacity, tone your muscles and firm the butt, thighs, and calves, and burn about 250 calories in half an hour of cycling.

Exercise bikes come in manual and electric versions. Manual versions are mostly used in spinning classes (see page 215), while electric versions have detailed exercise display information. The speed and resistance of an exercise bike can be adjusted to increase or decrease the difficulty of the ride, allowing you to burn more, or less, calories.

Some people prefer the comfort of a recumbent bike, which lets you ride with your legs extended horizontally. The reclined position engages the hamstrings and gets the quads to do the work, which relieves stress on your knees. Recumbent bikes are suitable for older people and those who are overweight or who have back problems.

Dance

Dancing strengthens bones and muscles, tones the entire body, improves balance, stamina, and flexibility, and reduces body tension. Dancing also has the advantage of being a fitness program that can easily be integrated into your social life. Try belly dancing's slides, twists, shimmies, and undulations to burn fat and condition your abs, hips, butts, thighs, and arms, and improve flexibility and posture. Be energized by fiery Latin dances—salsa, mambo, merengue, or zumba, a fusion of them all. Zumba routines combine fast and slow rhythms and utilize the principles of fitness interval training and resistance training to tone and sculpt the body.

DDR (Dance Dance Revolution)

DDR is a pioneering video game in a Japanese rhythm and dance series, and has become hugely popular since its release in 1999. Many American schools use DDR as part of fitness programs, and gyms make use of it, too, because the amount of active movement required to play DDR makes it a very effective, as well as fun, fat-burning aerobic exercise. Players stand on a "dance platform" or stage and hit colored arrows with their feet when prompted by quick-moving musical and visual cues. Players are judged by how well they time their dance to the patterns presented to them, and are allowed to choose more music to play to if they receive a passing score. You can play it in games arcades or buy a home version. Many home versions of the game have a workout mode to estimate calories burned and any changes in the player's weight.

Exercise machines

Exercise machines come in many shapes, styles, and sizes.

Cardio machines: A treadmill, probably the most familiar cardio machine, can be adapted to different fitness levels by increasing the speed from walking to running, and by adjusting the incline. Brisk walking on this machine burns about 100 calories per mile (about 60 calories per kilometer), making it the most efficient fat-burner of any cardio machines available at most gyms.

Elliptical machines and stair steppers: These are easier on the joints than a treadmill and because you use them in a standing position, you're working lots of muscles, so the calorie-burn rate is still high.

Resistance machines (see also resistance training): Resistance workout machines develop muscle and bone density by making your muscles produce extra force to overcome the resistance of the machine. The resistance can be provided by a series of cables, which pull up weight bars stacked on top of each other, or by hydraulics (air pressure), or by body weight. Different machines can be used to work the same muscle groups, depending on whether you are sitting, reclining, or standing. For example, the pulling exercise of a cable row machine is a great workout for the back, whereas a cable press machine targets your chest muscles.

Rowing machines: These provide an advanced cardiovascular workout using a lot of muscle groups. You need to engage your core abdominal muscles to support and protect your back, while you push with the legs and pull with the arms.

Stationary bikes: Of all exercise machines, these have the least impact on the joints. They are also less intense calorie-burners than other machines. You'll need to pedal four miles (six kilometers) to burn 100 calories.

Feldenkrais Method

The Feldenkrais Method teaches you how to move your body with less discomfort and greater ease than you were moving before. It is based on the recognition that our bodies tend to fall into habitual ways of moving, which cause more strain and tension than we realize. In Feldenkrais classes, the teacher gives directions to make you aware of the way you move your body, and suggests options for moving in a safer and more comfortable way.

In one-on-one sessions, your body absorbs a similar lesson through the gentle hands-on approach of a Feldenkrais practitioner. It can take between four and eight weeks to experience the effectiveness of the Feldenkrais Method, but the benefits are relief from tension and muscular pain, improved performance in physical activity, fuller breathing, and increased vitality.

Fencing

Fencing is a form of sword fighting, in which the object is to touch your opponent with the tip of the sword. The person with the most "hits" is the winner. It is an elegant, physically and mentally intense sport, and an effective fitness regimen. Fencing develops coordination, cardiovascular fitness, sharpened reflexes, muscle tone, poise, and confidence—and you'll probably do more squats and lunges than you would in an average aerobics class. A fencing match is made up of fights, or bouts, that can last up to 15 minutes. During that time, each fencer must attempt to score hits on their opponent.

High-intensity interval training

The principle of high-intensity interval training (HIIT) is that short intervals of maximum effort followed by longer intervals of low to moderate effort increase the number of calories you burn both during your exercise session and afterward. The calorie-burning continues because of the length of time it takes your body to recover from each session. You need to push yourself as hard as you possibly can during the high-intensity intervals, easing back somewhat during the moderate interludes to allow your body to replenish energy levels, but never stopping. So this is a particularly strenuous workout. Before starting any HIIT program, you should be able to exercise for at least 20 to 30 minutes at 70 to 85 percent of your estimated maximum heart rate, without feeling exhausted. HIIT is not for beginner exercisers or people with cardiovascular problems or risk factors.

Jogging

There is some debate about the difference between jogging and running. The simple answer is that jogging is just a slow form of running.

Some people say that any running that is recreational and not part of a training program should be called jogging. Others say that it's to do with mind-set. Calling yourself a "jogger" means you don't have the confidence to say you are a runner. Whether you are a slow runner or a jogger or a casual runner, the physical, social, and mental benefits of this cardiovascular exercise are tremendous.

Kickboxing

Kickboxing can be practiced for self-defence, sport, or fitness. It is a rigorous full-body aerobic and anaerobic workout that focuses on flexibility, hand/foot coordination, core strength, and cardio conditioning. Kickboxing can burn between 350 and 450 calories an hour and is a great stress reliever. No equipment is used and gloves are not required. You need to have a reasonable degree of fitness before you begin kickboxing classes.

Unlike other types of kickboxing, cardio kickboxing does not involve physical contact between competitors. Classes usually start with 10 to 15 minutes of warm-ups, followed by a 30-minute session that includes movements such as knee strikes, kicks, and punches. After this, at least five minutes should be devoted to cooling down, followed by about 10 minutes of stretching and muscle conditioning.

Exercise directory

Nia

This is a fusion fitness program that blends Korean martial art tae kwon do with tai chi, yoga, and dance. Its name is an acronym for non-impact aerobics, and also for neuromuscular integrative action. Classes are done barefoot to diverse and inspiring music with the aim of integrating the movement and concepts of the healing arts, the power and mindfulness of martial arts and meditative techniques, and the grace and expressiveness of dance techniques all in one cardiovascular workout.

Pilates

Named after Joseph Pilates, who first developed rehabilitation exercises for dancers, Pilates is a body conditioning system of more than 500 exercises that are designed to develop strength, flexibility, and postural awareness. Pilates works several muscle groups simultaneously through smooth, continuous motion, with a particular concentration on strengthening and stabilizing the body's core—the lower (deep) abdominal muscles and mid- and upper-back muscles.

Instruction is usually given in small group sessions by a qualified teacher. Movements aimed at improving strength, range of motion, coordination, balance, alignment, muscular symmetry, flexibility, and endurance are

performed on a floor mat and specially designed tables or chairs that use spring coil tension for resistance. The emphasis of Pilates on sustained stretches and close attention to form makes it very effective for injury prevention as well as rehabilitation.

Its eight guiding principles are relaxation, concentration, alignment, centering, breathing, coordination, flowing movements, and stamina.

Resistance training

Resistance training is any exercise that contracts the muscles against an external resistance in order to increase strength, tone, mass, and endurance. The external resistance can be provided by weights, hydraulic pressure, your own body weight, bricks, sandbags, or any object that causes the muscles to contract. Sometimes resistance training is referred to as "strength training," especially in regard to lifting weights.

Resistance training works by causing microscopic tears to the cells in your muscles, an effect referred to as "catabolism." The damaged muscle fiber is quickly repaired by the body as testosterone, growth hormone, protein, and other nutrients flood the cells and regenerate tissue. This process of regrowth, called "anabolism," is what strengthens muscles. Your muscles heal when you aren't working out, which is why it's necessary to leave time between workouts for recovery.

Resistance training is more effective the older we get, since it counters the inevitable decline of muscle fiber and helps to build bone density. It also helps to lower moderately high blood pressure and can raise metabolic weight, an important factor in maintaining a healthy body weight.

Running

A simple and satisfying fitness activity, running is accessible to anyone and that includes people in their 60s, 70s, and beyond. All you need is a pair of running shoes. Running strengthens the heart and bones, lowers blood pressure, boosts energy, and burns calories. When pursued out of doors, running invigorates the mind as well as the body. Most runners experience a feeling of wellbeing after a run, and a more positive mood. Some detractors say it is hard on the joints, particularly the knees, but wearing good shoes, being mindful of training levels, and varying the surfaces on which you run should prevent joint injury.

If you are starting a running routine from scratch, first you have to build up your stamina. Go for brisk walks and gradually, over days or weeks, increase the intensity of your pace. As you become accustomed to a harder workload, you can introduce jogging intervals into your routine. Power walk for a few minutes, and then jog for 30 seconds to a minute.

If your goal as a runner is to

enjoy yourself and stay healthy, you probably don't need to run for more than 30 or 40 minutes at a time. But if you want to push yourself, you can focus your training on a 5K race or half marathon, or even a full marathon. Training for a race is very motivational and gives you the opportunity to set a goal of running a personal best. Expect peaks and plateaus in your running as your body adapts to the demands you place on it. Be patient. Don't increase your workload in time or distance by more than 10 percent per week.

Running on a treadmill is an alternative to running outside when the weather is bad. Treadmill running can also be easier on your joints and requires less effort generally because of the lack of wind resistance. Most treadmills have controls that let you vary the pace and incline of the run. An incline setting of 1.5 percent simulates the wind resistance of running outdoors.

Spinning

Spinning is a high-intensity group workout on an exercise bike, and typically lasts anywhere from 30 to 75 minutes. It is a highly effective interval-training method for cardiovascular stamina and fat loss. Spinning bikes differ from regular stationary bikes in the way the wheels are connected to the pedals. If you stop pedaling on a spinning bike, the wheels and pedals will continue to move. Spinning bikes

resemble road bikes, with pedals into which you can clip your shoes.

Spinning classes use lights and music to create an exciting, energizing atmosphere. After a warm-up "ride," an instructor guides and motivates participants through workout phases that include sprint intervals, climbs, racing, and coasting, followed by a cool-down. You are encouraged to stand as you climb to work different muscles. You control resistance on your bike by using the gears to simulate climbing hills or racing downhill.

Swimming

Swimming is one of the most effective forms of aerobic exercise. While providing an allover body workout, it improves cardiovascular function, muscle strength, flexibility, and endurance. It's also great for weight loss—swimming at a medium intensity for 30 minutes will consume up to 200 calories—and at the same time is meditative and relaxing.

To get the most out of swimming, incorporate interval, speed, and endurance lengths. For variety, you can introduce different equipment and strokes to your workouts. Freestyle and backstroke tone the shoulders, arms, and stomach. Breaststroke tones thighs, stomach, and buttocks. Your stroke will be smoother, faster, and more efficient, if you breathe out when your face is underwater and breathe in as soon as your face is out of the water. Work up to using one breath for every

three strokes. The muscles you use most in swimming, especially in freestyle, are the latissimi dorsi, which extend down the sides of the back and up into the shoulder area. Always stretch them after a session while your muscles are still warm.

The support of the water greatly reduces stress on joints, such as knees and ankles. This makes swimming an ideal activity for people recovering from injury, those with back pain, arthritis, or other such conditions, older people, those carrying excess weight, and pregnant women.

Taoist martial arts

Taoist martial arts were developed by Chinese monks hundreds of years ago as methods of self-defence and ways of maintaining sound physical and mental health. These soft, or yin, styles of martial arts require physical fitness but not large muscles. They are safe practices for anyone from children to older people. Taoist practices tend to use circular movements and concentrate on developing and harnessing an individual's internal energy, known as "qi" or "chi," and sometimes referred to as the "life force."

There are numbers of different styles of each of these arts, but they all focus on cultivating suppleness, fitness, and correct breathing in order to attain inner calm and vitality. They boost the immune system by increasing blood circulation and releasing muscular tension. They improve digestion by strengthening and stimulating the nervous system, reduce emotional stress, and help relieve symptoms of fatigue and repetitive stress injuries.

Ba gua: This practice uses a constantly circling motion to follow the ebb and flow of yin and yang energies. The focus on balance and fluidity coupled with gentle, low-impact movements makes this an ideal style for promoting healing. Many tai chi schools incorporate ba gua in their training.

Qigong: Qigong employs slow, fluid postures synchronized with the breath, meditation, and self-massage, to expand and concentrate the circulation of qi in the body. Qigong breathing practices are often used to prepare for tai chi exercises, but qigong can be performed separately.

Tai chi: Tai chi is a series of gentle, deliberate movements, performed so that the body flows smoothly from one position to another in a set sequence. Each series is called a "form" and each form contains between 20 and 100 moves, and requires up to 20 minutes to complete. The names of forms are derived from nature—for example, "Wave Hands Like Clouds," or "Grasping the Bird's Tail." In order to balance yin and yang, the movements are practiced in pairs of opposites. For example, a turn to the right follows one to the left. While doing these exercises, you are urged to pay close attention to your breathing, which is centered in the diaphragm.

Tai chi emphasizes technique rather than strength or power, although the slow, precise movements require good muscle control. Meditative concentration is focused on a point just below the navel, from which it is believed qi radiates throughout the body.

Tai chi is taught in many health clubs, schools, and recreational facilities. Practitioners believe that daily sessions are needed in order to get the most benefit. Once you have mastered a form, you can practice it at home.

Walking

Walking is the simplest exercise you can undertake to lower blood pressure, but for it to be effective you have to walk at a reasonably energetic pace rather than just strolling. Fitness walking (sometimes called power walking) involves using a purposeful stride, arms pumping, heart rate increased. This vigorous style helps to burn fat, reduce bone loss, and tone muscles in the buttocks, thighs, hips, shoulders, upper back, and abs. Walking is easy on the joints, since you hit the ground with less than half the force you do when you run.

Aim for four to six fitness walks per week, each lasting from 20 to 30 minutes. Try to increase your walking by 10 percent per week. If you're currently walking for 30 minutes per day on four days each week, that means adding just 12 minutes to your total weekly walking time.

Yoga

Yoga is among the oldest known systems of exercise in the world, practiced for physical and mental health, and spiritual wellbeing. The combination of physical postures, breathing exercises, and meditation techniques has been shown to reduce stress, lower blood pressure, regulate heart rate, and even slow down the aging process. Yoga, in common with other mind/body practices, such as tai chi and qigong, encourages an increasingly calm mental state as the body intensifies its muscular work. Yoga postures (or asanas) involve the repeated contraction and relaxation of large muscle groups, which signal the brain to release specific neurotransmitters that make you feel simultaneously relaxed and more receptive. You can practice yoga anywhere, including sitting in a chair.

There are many different forms of yoga, including slow-paced styles, such as hatha and yin yoga, and others of more physical intensity. The latter usually employ "vinyasa," which means "breath-synchronized movement," to progress from one pose to the next. This technique is sometimes referred to as "vinyasa flow" because of the smooth way that the poses run together and become like a dance. Vinyasa styles are anusara, ashtanga, Bikram (hot), jivamukti, kundalini, and power yoga.

Anusara: The meaning of anusara is "flowing with grace." The "three As" of this style are Attitude, Alignment, and Action. Anusara classes are based on a philosophy of intrinsic goodness and emphasize heart-opening through backbending. The classes include vinyasa flow and use props to achieve correct alignment.

Ashtanga: This style of yoga is athletic and physically demanding, focusing on a set series of poses that are performed in a flowing vinyasa style. There are six different series of advancing difficulty, although realistically most practitioners only ever complete the first, or primary, series, and the second, or intermediate series.

The primary series aims to realign the spine, detoxify the body, and build strength, flexibility, and stamina. The series consists of about 75 poses. They take an hour and a half to two hours to complete, beginning with Sun Salutations and moving on to standing poses, seated poses, inversions, and backbends, followed by cool-down exercises.

Bikram (hot) yoga: Bikram yoga follows a specific 26-posture (or asana) sequence, and is practiced in a room that is heated to 100°F (38°C) in order to make the body more flexible. You will need your own yoga mat and towel for a Bikram class, since you will be sweating so much. Students tend to wear very little clothing for the same reason.

Hatha yoga: Although most forms of yoga that employ specific postures are technically "hatha," this term is generally used for slow-paced classes that include some simple breathing exercises and perhaps seated meditation as well as performing the postures. A hatha class is a good place to learn basic postures and relaxation techniques.

Iyengar yoga: A methodical style, Iyengar yoga focuses on the anatomical precision of each posture. Props, including belts and bolsters, are used to assist with proper alignment. Postures in an Iyengar class are often held for long periods of time with the emphasis on the posture's quality of expression. Iyengar yoga came to the United States in 1974.

Jivamukti: Derived from ashtanga yoga, jivamukti means "liberation while living." Each class has a theme, which is explored through postures, Sanskrit, chanting, music, and meditation.

Kundalini: This is one of the more spiritual types of yoga. It goes beyond the physical performance of poses with its emphasis on breathing, meditation, and chanting. Kundalini sequences (called kriyas) may consist of rapid, repetitive movements synchronized with the breath, or holding a pose while breathing in a particular way. The sequences look simple but are physically very intense.

Power yoga: Based on ashtanga, but less traditional, power yoga is a strong, continuously moving practice that builds endurance and strength, and allows you to sweat tension out of the body.

Yin yoga: A calm practice, yin yoga cultivates a deep sense of awareness by holding gentle poses, often supported by props, for a long time. The prolonged, supported holding of the pose aims to release deep tension in the muscles and connective tissues, and promotes physical, mental, and emotional openness and flexibility.

Citations

Chapter 1

"Breast cancer preventable if lifestyle changes are made": World Cancer Research Fund review, September 2009.

"Relation between modifiable lifestyle factors and lifetime risk of heart failure": *Journal of the American Medical Association*, 2009.

"Diet and lifestyle risk factors associated with incident hypertension in women": *Journal of the American Medical Association*, 2009

"UK obesity": *Journal of Epidemiology and Community Health*, December 2008.

"American obesity in 2015": Study by Johns Hopkins Bloomberg School of Public Health, *Epidemiologic Review*, August 2007.

"Australian obesity": Access Economics Report for *Diabetes Australia*, August 2008.

"Vigorous exercise in middle age will help you to live longer": *Annals of Internal Medicine*, August 2008.

"Fit body, Fit mind? Forestall decline in cognitive function and reduce risk of dementia": Scientific American Mind, July/August 2009.

Fit For Life: Ranulph Fiennes, Little Brown, 1999.

Galloway's Book on Running: Jeff Galloway, Shelter Publications, 2002.

Chapter 2

"Angina: More Evidence for the Benefit of Exercise in Cardiovascular Disease—and Even in Heart Failure": European Society of Cardiology, May 2009.

"Aerobic training using a cycloergometer improved the physical capacity of cardiac patients": Dr Tomasz Mikulski, Medical Research Center in Warsaw, Poland.

"Walking on a cobblestone mat surface results in significant reductions in blood pressure": Oregon Research Institute, *Journal of the American Geriatrics Society*, 2005.

"Intense exercise is better than moderate exercise for lowering cholesterol": Duke University Medical Center, 2002.

"Exercise slows progression of peripheral arterial disease": *Annals of Internal Medicine*, January 2009.

"Patients with arterial disease and hospital-supervised exercise": *The Journal of Physiology*, December 2008.

"People who are physically active before suffering a stroke recover better": *Journal of the American Academy of Neurology*, October 2008.

Chapter 3

"Indoor and outdoor cycling reduces the frequency of attacks": *Headache: The Journal of Head and Face Pain*, April 2009.

"People living with multiple sclerosis report exercise improves their fatigue levels": Everydayhealth.com

"Moderate regular exercise helps to correct bladder control issues that are common in people with multiple sclerosis": *Inside MS*, Fall 1995.

"Nintendo Wii May Enhance Parkinson's Treatment": Medical College of Georgia, June 2009.

Chapter 4

"An Angry Heart Can Lead To Sudden Death": *Journal of the American College of Cardiology*, March 2009.

"The effect of exercise on clinical depression and depression resulting from mental illness: a meta-analysis": *Journal of Clinical Psychiatry* 6(3), 2004.

Anger Kills: Redford Williams, Random House, 1994.

"Kundalini Yoga Stretch Pose": *The Eight Human Talents*: Gurmukh, HarperResource, 2000.

"Ecotherapy: the green agenda for mental health": Mind, June 2009.

"Integrating physical activity into mental health services for persons with serious mental illness": *Psychiatric Services* 56(3), 2005.

"The effects of exercise therapy on clients in a psychotic rehabilitation program": *Psychosocial Rehabilitation Journal* 16, 1993.

"Fitness: A visible adjunct to treatment for young adults with psychiatric disabilities": *Psychosocial Rehabilitation Journal* 15(3), 1992.

"Schizophrenia and weight management: A systematic review of interventions to control weight": *Acta Psychiatry Scandinavian* 108(5), 2003.

Exercise, health and mental health: emerging relationships: Edited by Guy E.J. Faulkner, Adrian H. Taylor, Routledge, 2005.

"Spinning for Psychosis" in "Coming Off Psychiatric Medication": www.comingoff.com

Wellness and Fitness in Recovery: Benefits of Exercise in Promoting Sobriety Maintenance and Optimal Health": *Counselor, The Magazine for Addiction Professionals*, April 2006.

"The Role of a Physical Fitness

Programme in the Treatment of Alcoholism": *Journal of Studies on Alcohol* 43, no. 3, 1982.

"Acute exercise modulates cigarette cravings and brain activation in response to smoking-related images": *Psychopharmacology*, 2008.

"Exercise has been shown to help protect the brain against addiction," says Mark A. Smith, a professor of neuroscience at Davidson University. His research on rats shows that access to exercise reduces the appeal of cocaine.

"Running and Addiction: Precipitated Withdrawal in a Rat Model of Activity-Based Anorexia": *Behavioral Neuroscience*, August 2009.

"Could Exercise Regenerate Alcohol-Damaged Neurons?" *Psychiatry News*, December 2006.

Chapter 5

Guidelines for the Diagnosis and Management of Asthma: National Heart, Lung, and Blood Institute, US Dept of Health and Human Services, NIH publications 08-40512007.

"Athletes With Asthma Need More Help From Their Team Trainers": *Science Daily*, Ohio State University, April 2009.

"Exercise Improves Cardiopulmonary Fitness In Asthma": Center for the Advancement of Health, October 2005.

"Regular exercise can help people with COPD reduce anxiety and depression, and improve endurance and some kinds of intellectual functioning": *Health Psychology*, May 1998.

Chapter 6

"Tai chi relieves pain and disability among people with arthritis": *Arthritis Care & Research*, June 2009.

"A randomized controlled trial of tai chi for long-term low back pain (TAI CHI): Study rationale, design, and methods": *BMC Musculoskeletal Disorders* 10 (1), 2009.

"Working with weights provides relief for people with back pain": *Journal of Strength and Conditioning Research*, 2009.

"Alexander technique lessons in combination with an exercise programme offer long-term effective treatment for chronic back pain": online *British Medical Journal*, April 2008.

"Evaluation of the Effectiveness and Efficacy of Iyengar Yoga Therapy on Chronic Low Back Pain": *Spine*, September 2009.

"Muscle strengthening exercises for low back pain": Robert J. Daul, MPT www.spine-health.com/wellness/exercise

"Exercise in warm water decreases pain and improves cognitive function in middle-aged women with fibromyalgia": *Clinical and Experimental Rheumatology*, Nov–Dec 2007.

"Benefits of pool-based exercise for people with fibromyalgia": *Arthritis & Rheumatism*, February 2001.

"Qigong is as effective as exercise therapy for alleviating long-term, nonspecific neck pain": *Spine*, October 2007.

"Lean body mass and weight-bearing activity in the prediction of bone mineral density in physically active men": *Journal of Strength Conditioning*, February 2009.

"Leisure physical activity and the risk of fracture in men": *PLoS Med* 4(6), 2007.

Yoga: The Path to Holistic Health: B.K.S. Iyengar (Dorling Kindersley, London 2001). Photos and detailed descriptions of poses for the relief of sciatica.

Chapter 7

"People who engage in frequent physical exercise experience fewer symptoms of GERD": *Gut*, 2004.

"Excess body weight increases risk of GERD": *The American Journal of Gastroenterology*, 2004.

"Prevalence of irritable bowel syndrome, influence of lifestyle factors and bowel habits in Korean college students": *International Journal of Nursing Studies* 42, 2005.

"A randomized trial of yoga for adolescents with irritable bowel syndrome": *Pain Research & Management*, 2006: 217–223.

"Runners' diarrhea: Different patterns and associated factors": *Journal of Clinical Gastroenterology* 14, 1992.

Chapter 8

"Even Modest Exercise Can Reduce Negative Effects Of Belly Fat": *American Journal of Physiology, Endocrinology, and Metabolism*, April 2009.

"Tai chi and qigong prompt significant improvement in blood glucose levels and metabolic syndrome": *British Journal of Sports Medicine*, December 2008.

"Effects of Aerobic Training, Resistance Training, or Both on Glycemic Control in Type 2 Diabetes: A Randomized Trial": *Annals of Internal Medicine*, September 2007.

"Comparison of Combined Aerobic and High-Force Eccentric Resistance Exercise with Aerobic Exercise only for People with Type 2 Diabetes Mellitus": *Physical Therapy*, 2008.

"Visceral fat adipokine secretion is associated with systemic inflammation in obese humans": *Diabetes*, published online, February 7, 2007.

"Belly Fat may Drive Inflammatory Processes Associated with Disease": Washington University School of Medicine, March 2007.

"Six sessions of sprint interval training increases muscle oxidative potential and cycle endurance capacity in humans": *Journal of Applied Physiology* 98: 1985–1990, February 2005.

"Effect of an acute period of resistance exercise on excess post-exercise oxygen consumption: implications for body mass management": *Journal of Applied Physiology*, March 2002.

"Two weeks of high-intensity aerobic interval training increases the capacity for fat oxidation during exercise in women": *Journal of Applied Physiology*, December 2006.

"A Healthy Mix of Rest and Motion": *The New York Times*, Peter Jaret, May 3, 2007.

Chapter 9

"Fire breathing instructions for liver congestion": *Theories of the Chakras*: Hiroshi Motoyama, *New Age Books*, 1981.

"Weight Loss Reduces Incontinence In Obese Women": University of California, San Francisco, February 2009.

"Pelvic Floor Muscle Exercises can help Manage Urinary Incontinence in Older Women": Rush University Medical Center, October 2009.

Chapter 10

"Chronic Insomnia as a Risk Factor for Developing Anxiety and Depression": *Sleep*, July 2009.

"Meditation May be an Effective Treatment For Insomnia": American Academy of Sleep Medicine, June 2009.

"Insomnia is Bad for the Heart; Increases Blood Pressure": University of Montreal, September 2009.

"Moderate Exercise can improve Sleep Quality of Insomnia Patients": American Academy of Sleep Medicine, June 2008.

"Exercise training effect on obstructive sleep apnea syndrome": Sleep Res Online, 3: 2000.

"Effects of Oropharyngeal Exercises on Patients with Moderate Obstructive Sleep Apnea" and "Association of Physical Activity with Sleep-Disordered Breathing": *Sleep Breath*, 24, 2007.

"How to strengthen your palate and tongue to help snoring and obstructive apnoea": South Devon Healthcare NHS Trust.

Chapter 11

Turning Point: The Myths and Realities of Menopause: C. Sue Furman, Oxford University Press, 1995 (p.72 Sex as a remedial activity.)

"Women who regularly engage in any physical activity are 31% less likely to develop diabetes": *American Journal of Public Health*, January 2000.

"Exercise benefits skin": *Ending Aging: The Rejuvenation Breakthroughs that Could Reverse Human Aging in our Lifetime*: Aubrey de Grey with Michael Rae, St Martins Press, 2007.

Women, Hormones and the Menstrual Cycle: Ruth Trickey, Allen & Unwin, 1998.

"Effect of a Synthetic Progestin on the Exercise Status of Sedentary Young Women": *The Journal of Clinical Endocrinology & Metabolism* Vol. 90, 2005.

"Effects of Maternal Exercise on the Fetal Heart": Findings presented at the 121st annual meeting of the American Physiological Society, part of the Experimental Biology 2008 scientific conference.

Chapter 12

"Forestall decline in cognitive function and reduce risk of dementia": Fit Body, Fit Mind? Scientific American Mind, July/August 2009.

"Evidence-based Tai Chi program to prevent falls among older adults": *American Journal of Public Health*, July 2008.

"Endurance improves as you age": *Exercise and Sports Sciences Reviews*, January 2009.

"Exercise, Longevity and Life Expectancy": Mark Stibich, About.com

"The Association between Physical Activity in Leisure Time and Leukocyte Telomere Length": *Annals of Internal Medicine* 168(2), 2008.

"Regular exercise may reduce the risk of dementia and Alzheimer's disease in the elderly by as much as 40%": *Annals of Internal Medicine* 144, 2005.

"Incidence and etiology of dementia in a large elderly Italian population":

Neurology, May 2005.

"A prospective study of walking as compared with vigorous exercise in the prevention of coronary heart disease in women": *The New England Journal of Medicine*, August 1999.

"Weight training improves walking endurance in healthy elderly persons": *Annals of Internal Medicine*, March 1996.

"Balance exercises reduce seniors' risk of falling": *Journal of the American Geriatrics Society*, December 2008

Chapter 13

"Strenuous exercise for 30 minutes every day can halve the chance of dying from cancer": *British Journal of Sports Medicine*, 2009.

"Intensity and timing of physical activity in relation to postmenopausal breast cancer risk": *BMC Cancer*, 2009.

"Exercise and Rest Reduce Cancer Risk": American Association for Cancer Research, November 2008.

"Physical activity and colon cancer prevention: a meta-analysis": *British Journal of Cancer*, 2009.

Index

INDEX

Acknowledgments

Sequence photography
Thanks to models Liz Westlake, Jessie Miller, and Cathy Tinknell; and MOT models Gregg, Jason, Joanne, and Kali. Particular thanks to personal trainer Lucy Wyndham Read (pages 120, 132, 164, 165; www.lucywyndhamread.com) and Pilates instructor Anya Wilson (pages 128–129, 190–191).